Handbook of staff development

A practical guide for health professionals

Barbara Horner

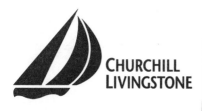

CHURCHILL
LIVINGSTONE

CHURCHILL LIVINGSTONE
An imprint of Pearson Professional

Pearson Professional (Australia) Pty Ltd
Kings Gardens, 95 Coventry Street, South Melbourne 3205 Australia

Copyright © Pearson Professional (Australia) Pty Ltd 1995
First published 1995

National Library of Australia Cataloguing-in-Publication Data

Horner, Barbara Joan.
    Handbook of staff development: a practical guide for
    health professionals

    Includes index.
    ISBN 0 443 05145 3.

    1. Employees – Training of – Handbooks, manuals, etc.
    2. Public health personnel – In-service training – Handbooks,
    manuals, etc. I. Title

610.7307155

Editing: Pam Jonas
Indexing: Max McMaster
Produced by Churchill Livingstone in Melbourne
Printed in Australia

The
publisher's
policy is to use
**paper manufactured
from sustainable forests**

Contents

Introduction

Health care is a unique and complex business. Like all other businesses, a health care organisation must function with the resources that are available, financial, physical and human; and within the boundaries imposed by economic and political constraints. Health care in the 1990s is a competitive business.

Health care is also a people business—people deliver the service and people experience what is delivered. In the delivery of health care there is a demand for high performance and high commitment from the health care providers, the human resources of the organisation. The nature of the business provides little opportunity for error and expectations are high.

This book is based upon the belief that in all organisations, including health care organisations, an investment in the human resources will make the most significant difference to the performance of the organisation. Health care moves through phases of scientific and technological change and development. In recent years, political and economic pressures have forced health care organisations to review their structures, functions, procedures and outcomes. Through all of this, one thing remains constant—the human resources of the organisation, the people who deliver the health care. Because they are always there, there is a risk that they will be taken for granted, under valued or ignored. The people hold the organisation together.

An organisation needs to recognise that an investment in staff development will move an organisation from acceptable performance to excellent performance. No matter how tight the budget, how rigid the constraints, staff development cannot be sacrificed.

This book brings together knowledge and practical experience from a career of many years working with people. It is a practical, useful book that presents knowledge, application, personal experience and real examples. It aims to assist those who are in a staff development role and those who hold responsibility for the management of staff development. It is, however, a book that can be used by anyone in an organisation who has a commitment to improving performance.

The book can be used in different ways. Ideally, it should be read from the beginning to end, for then the information will be read in a logical and meaningful sequence. Every chapter, however, stands alone and so the reader can begin the book at any chapter, to seek out specific information or for a specific purpose. Within the book, some text has been emphasised to either indicate important information, or to highlight a practical example. Each chapter begins with questions to assist the reader to recognise the content and to guide their learning. References are given for each chapter and further resources are provided in Chapter 9. The book is learner-centred. It is for you to determine how best to use the book and to apply the information. These examples show how the book can be used:

You are recently appointed to a staff development position and have been advised that a staff needs assessment is required. Where do you begin? Chapter 2 provides an explanation of needs assessment.

You are a divisional manager and you hold responsibility for all activities within your division. You have no qualifications or experience in education and, in terms of staff development, you do not know where to begin. Chapter 1 provides an explanation of the staff development process.

You are a senior manager involved in a review and restructuring program that includes a review of all organisational departments. The review is considering appointing a staff development co-ordinator. Chapter 8 provides guidelines for selecting someone for a position in staff de–velopment.

Finally, this book presents education as a life long process of learning. For the individual, learning never ends. For the organisation, learning must be the reason for all change. An organisation with a commitment to learning will recognise the importance of staff development and will implement a staff development process in recognition of the importance of their human resources. This book will guide that process.

The concept of staff development

Key questions

- What is the difference between staff development, continuing education and inservice?

- What is the relationship between staff development and human resource management?

- Who is responsible for staff development — employer or employee?

- What are the components of staff development?

Content summary

Introduction

Employers, such as health care agencies, academic institutions and large companies, recognise that a relationship exists between organisational effectiveness and productivity and staff satisfaction. Organisational effectiveness and productivity should improve in a system which allows for the maximum utilisation of the employee's knowledge and skills. This realisation may result in the establishment of a staff development unit or the allocation of specific responsibilities for staff development to an individual as part of a job description or position statement.

Staff development in the work place is no longer an option. Maximum performance can not be achieved, nor productivity realised without a commitment to staff development. Health care today demands excellence in performance and a high quality of service, where service refers to the care that is being delivered. Such high standards can be achieved only if the human resources, that is the staff of the organisation, are considered as important as either the physical or financial resources.

Staff development is a process that should occur as part of a contractual employment relationship between an employer and an employee. Learning as a life long process is well illustrated in health care where the need to adapt to change is constant, with technological developments, changes to role and responsibility, varying economic and political demands, changes to funding and increasing public awareness and expectation of quality service.

Every individual brings skills, knowledge and personal attributes to a position, which may have been identified as specific for that position. But learning about that position and the environment in which they will work, begins from the time of employment and continues throughout employment. A clearly identified process of staff development will assist the individual to move along this continuum of learning.

This chapter will discuss the meaning of staff development and define common terms. It will discuss the relationship between staff development and human resource management, a model for a staff development process, a framework for staff development and the need for a strong relationship between employer and employee.

The meaning of staff development

Definitions of staff development vary, as do explanations of the responsibilities of a staff development department. Other commonly used terms, such as continuing education and inservice, describe components of the role, but are not sufficiently comprehensive to address the full scope of responsibilities.

Continuing education has been defined as planned organised experiences that are designed to meet specific learning needs and objectives (Gathers 1988), or as the formal study undertaken to extend or update knowledge, or to meet advances or changes of direction in a career (Streatfield 1987 in Brennan 1990). Inservice can be described as planned education programs provided by an employer for employees in an organisation to maintain and/or update skills and knowledge relevant to a work or employment context (Gathers 1988).

There has also been considerable debate over the difference between training and education. Training implies the acquisition of certain skills, whereas education implies the acquisition of skills, knowledge and attitudes which requires further understanding and aims to bring about a change in behaviour. These terms are often used interchangeably or both at the same time without recognising this difference in depth of understanding. In most cases, the expected outcome of training is not the same as that of education.

Clearly, all these terms will have different meaning for different people. Arguing over the definitions is an interesting intellectual exercise at best but it is the application that is really important. In this book I use the term staff development and define it in this way:

Definition of staff development

A planned and organised process of learning within an employment setting, designed to update or increase knowledge and/or skills or for personal growth and development, to improve performance or to meet advances or changes in direction or focus of a position or of an organisation.

Staff development is about much more than just how to do a job. It requires a commitment to the development of the whole person. Rather than focus on definitions of terms, it is more useful to examine staff development in terms of the needs that staff identify.

Research has identified that staff development needs can be classified into three key areas (Horner 1990). They are:

- the need for knowledge and skills for a specific position
- the need for job satisfaction
- the need for positive interpersonal relationships.

The need for knowledge and skills for a specific position

All jobs require skills and knowledge, sometimes expressed as qualifications and expertise, or qualifications and experience, which should be stated clearly within the job description/position statement. In some cases, minimum performance standards are also set; for example, competencies for the beginning nursing practitioner as determined for registration. These are not usually stated in the job description but addressed within the requirement of registration. In some cases specific qualifications are required, for example, a degree in a discipline. In other cases specific experience is identified; for example, a number of years in a similar position with similar responsibilities. Selection should consider knowledge and skills for the current position as well as an anticipated role in the future with an expansion of service, change in technology or reorganisation of responsibilities. In other words, astute selection should focus on present and future needs.

No position remains the same for ever and an organisation that is growing and changing, should anticipate that an individual will need to acquire new knowledge and learn new skills. An organisation where nothing changes will be left behind in the market place and the employees are likely to become bored and/or complacent. Employers who plan for growth and development will recognise that staff will need different knowledge and skills as the organisation or service changes. An effective staff development program will be aware of both the needs of the organisation as well as those of the individual and will plan to address both within a program.

There is always so much to know in any job and it can be difficult to identify all the knowledge and skills required. In health care knowledge and skills can be grouped into categories.

- Knowledge and skills specific to the client population:
    socio-economic characteristics
    treatment rates and classifications
    cultural groupings and patterns
    case-mix or funding classifications
    community needs for health care services.
- Knowledge and skills relating to clinical practice:
    clinical procedures or conditions
    advances in technology and changes in treatment
    legislative requirements of practice
    legal and ethical responsibilities.
- Knowledge and skills not specific to the client population or clinical practice:
    health care policy
    research methodology
    industrial relations
    organisational policy and procedures
    personnel procedures
    budgeting.

Categories like these three can assist staff and organisations to identify specific needs. They may provide direction for data collection and may become the basis of future programs. It is also important to recognise that broad categories of knowledge and skill may stay the same, but levels of expertise required may change or additional information may be needed within a specific area of knowledge or for a specific skill. On the other hand, new knowledge or skills may be required to meet new situations.

With the appointment of the very best person for a position, the employer should be assured that the individual has the knowledge, skill and experience for the position. Over time, however, the position is sure to change to meet the needs of the client population or the organisation. The individual will develop new needs or more advanced needs. Effective staff development will anticipate these changing needs.

The need for job satisfaction

Levine (1983) describes job satisfaction as comprising factors that focus on attitudinal responses to the job and refers to them as quality of work life factors; that is, those factors that make a difference to the employee and how he/she feels about a job. It is sometimes difficult for an individual to describe how he/she obtains job satisfaction, as job dissatisfaction, is often easier to recognise. But every individual knows how it feels to feel good about a job. An individual who feels good about a job looks forward to coming to work, whereas the individual who does not feel good about a job may work only for days off. If you work Monday to Friday, ask yourself the question, Do you come to work for Monday morning or Friday afternoon? (Are your days off the best part of your job?) The answer is a good measure of how much you enjoy your job, or, as Levine would say, a measure of your perception of the quality of your work life.

Employees who enjoy their job will produce better results so, in terms of staff development, it is valuable to identify what creates and what diminishes job satisfaction, so that gaps can be identified and needs can be met. Factors contributing to job satisfaction (quality of work life) in health care have been identified as falling into three areas (Horner 1990). Staff may need development in one or all of these areas and the astute employer will identify what is needed to increase the level of job satisfaction. Satisfied employees stay longer, work harder, appear committed, initiate change and progress. On the other hand, dissatisfied employees leave when they find something better, just do the job, give the bare minimum and often ignore or resist change.

Factors contributing to job satisfaction fall into three areas:

- Processes relating to personnel functions:
    the selection process and initial appointment
    opportunities for career advancement and growth
    work practices that encourage delegation and responsibility
    performance appraisal processes and practices
    lines and levels of communication.
- Interaction with clients:
    opportunities for effective communication
    relationships with clients/relatives/friends
    the opportunity to empower clients to take control of their situation
    feedback that you, the individual, have made a difference and contributed to the outcome of care.
- Factors contributing to the management of the role:
    management and control of work load on a daily basis
    the opportunity for planning and problem solving
    feelings towards and relationships with management staff
    perceptions of making a contribution to, and being important to, the team
    the opportunity for autonomous, independent practice
    the existence and availability of support.

The employer, and often staff in management positions, may only see staff development as related to the client population and their needs, and seek results from staff development in terms of improvements in client service. Factors that contribute to an individual's job satisfaction are just as important to the individual, but unfortunately they are often overlooked. The employee who is feeling satisfied about a job will automatically work towards client satisfaction and an improvement in service.

The need for positive interpersonal relationships

Interaction with people is a key aspect of health care as health care is a people business. A successful outcome in health care is often measured by the nature of the interaction between client and health care worker. Health care workers often work as part of a team, so that relationships with colleagues are also very important. It is often assumed that people know how to get on with each other, but unfortunately this is not always the case. The nature of health care often results in potentially difficult or uncomfortable situations where the interaction can cause considerable distress to client and/or worker.

Effective interpersonal relationships are an art, and an investment in assisting individuals to improve their ability to interact can pay huge dividends to the employer. Some of the needs that might be identified in this area are:

- assertive behaviour
- effective communication
- conflict resolution
- problem solving
- dealing with stressful situations
- leadership and delegation.

Many factors contribute to interpersonal relationships and multiple needs may be identified. One factor may relate to self health and needs might be identified in physical and emotional health status, self concept or self esteem, coping mechanism (dealing with difficult situations), or balancing work and personal/family commitments and responsibilities. A second factor may relate to career needs and needs may be identified in the ability to plan a career, study effectively, set goals, apply for promotion or a new position, or dealing with retirement, redundancy or dismissal. A third factor may relate to communication and might identify needs in assertive behaviour, public speaking, nonverbal communication, listening skills or documentation.

Individuals will have difficulty focusing on other areas of staff development if their personal needs are not met. No matter how important a new clinical skill may be, it will be difficult to give it full attention if the individual is feeling upset, frustrated or angry over an interaction with a client or colleague.

In summary then, staff development should be a process of learning that commences when an individual is employed and continues throughout the entire period of employment. Staff development needs are often identified in three key areas: factors that relate to knowledge and skills for a specific position, factors that contribute to job satisfaction and factors that contribute to positive interpersonal interaction.

Staff development is multifaceted and involves far more than just how to do a job. It is more than inservice and continuing education and requires a commitment to the development of the whole person.

Staff development and human resource management

Human resource management can be seen as a positive reflection of the move of the personnel department to a more central place in an organisation, with a presumption that the human resources of an organisation are considered equal to other resources. Horsefield (1988) describes human resource management as a strategic function, influenced by the culture and values of an organisation; whereas personnel management is primarily an operational and tactical activity concerned with organisational maintenance. This means that the purpose of human resource management is tied to the goals and purpose of an entire organisation.

Human resource management

The goal of corporate policy in human resources should be to develop a creative, proactive approach to organisational development. The purposes of human resource management (Donovan & Jackson 1991) can be described in five ways:

- improvement of the organisation's productivity by influencing the utilisation of the work force, the establishment of a human resource philosophy and by practices within the organisation
- enhancement of the quality of work life of the organisation, through communication pathways and strategies that facilitate two-way com—munication
- compliance with all the necessary laws and regulations relating to utilisation of human resources, such as health and safety, freedom of information, equal opportunity, sex discrimination
- development of industrial relations policies and practices
- development of communication and consultation within and between all levels of the organisation

Such purposes can only be achieved with good planning and it is within this planning that the importance of staff development becomes obvious. Human resource planning may be seen to comprise four key components. Staff development features in all components:

1 The acquisition of human resources, including the analysis of requirements, recruitment, selection, familiarisation and orientation.
2 The development of human resources, including career planning, performance appraisal and staff development (training or education programmes).

3 The maintenance of human resources, including attention to quality of work life factors, rewards, promotion, change and job enrichment.
4 The renewal of human resources, which might include retirement counselling, redundancy management and replacement.

Human resource management and staff development

Human resource management recognises the importance of staff development and human resource departments may allocate specific staff development functions or activities. Alternatively, there may be a specific section within the department with responsibility for all staff development functions or activities. Staff development can be approached in a number of different ways (Donovan and Jackson 1991) within the human resource management approach.

Approaches to staff development

Individual approach:
Staff development is linked closely to individual needs and aspirations through an appraisal approach where needs relating to job rotation and courses can be identified.
Results oriented approach:
Needs are identified, options ranked and the results evaluated in terms of measurable outcomes through a problem-solving approach; it focuses on short term needs.
Human resource planning approach:
The organisation develops its own training capability and this implies a degree of confidence in the organisation's ability to anticipate the future adequately; training fits in within a corporate management approach.

There has been a move toward decentralised management in health care organisations in recent years. This often results in the devolution of human resource management, and subsequently staff development responsibilities, to departments or areas. This move may be seen to facilitate the identification of individual or department needs and to promote concepts of delegation and empowerment. In terms of staff development there are positive outcomes of this style of management. Individual departments can organise their own staff development to meet specific needs, staff can feel a greater sense of ownership of their development and local strategies can allow more flexibility and accommodate local constraints.

However, there are also negative outcomes for this approach. A centralised department can ensure that the company mission and objectives are reinforced, some standardisation of strategies is more likely, and staff development does not get lost in day to day management issues and priorities. With the very best intentions in the world, if priorities change, resources are reallocated, or day to day management demands alter, staff development plans will be dropped. This rarely happens in a centralised system. In a decentralised system, however staff development will always be sacrificed to other needs or demands perceived to be more important at the time.

Staff development process

It can be seen that staff development is a complex phenomenon which can best be understood by viewing it as an ongoing process of activities. This approach helps to break down staff development into manageable chunks or stages which can be viewed from an individual or an organisational perspective. The responsibilities for someone working in staff development and the resources needed to establish a staff development department or to develop a staff development strategy are then more easily recognised. (For discussion of strategies see Ch. 3.)

An individual begins a relationship with an organisation from the first inquiry about a position. In fact, the wording of an advertisement can have a significant impact on early impressions and can encourage or discourage an individual to apply. Therefore, the first stage is recruitment. A judgement is made on the recruitment strategies to be used in terms of information that is presented, how a position is marketed, and against a clear statement of the qualifications and/or experience required. This identifies the importance of clear job descriptions and clear information for applicants.

The second stage of the process involves the selection of an individual for a specific position. When planning for selection, it is necessary to decide what tools to use, who to involve, the criteria for selection, and to set the scene for the development of a positive relationship between parties. There are many tools that can be used and selection will be enhanced by a composite package of tools. For example, a curriculum vitae or resume, references, interview process, practical examples, testing and problem solving scenarios are all ways to find out as much information as possible to aid in making the best decision.

The third stage results in an actual appointment and can be seen as part of the selection process. However, by making appointment a separate stage, the importance of establishing the initial connection to the organisation is recognised. At this time the new employee is making a commitment to the organisation by accepting a job offer and the organisation is acknowledging a commitment to the employee by accepting responsibility to assimilate the individual into the organisation. These first three stages can be recognised as significant personnel functions within the staff development role.

Now the process moves into the stages more readily recognised as education or inservice.

The fourth stage is orientation which can be described as the process of introducing an individual to the philosophy, goals, procedures, role expectations, facilities and services of an organisation and in relation to a specific position. It includes a process of socialisation through which the employee acquires attributes, norms and practices of employment. The length of time in this stage can vary from perhaps two weeks to three months, dependant on the complexity of the position, and can consist of a variety of activities and educational strategies. It is essential that performance expectations are clear at this stage and it has been found to be most useful if the new employee establishes a relationship with a buddy or preceptor. One of the most significant characteristics of this stage is that the new employee is given permission to be a learner and to ask questions and should therefore not be expected to perform at an unrealistic level of expertise.

The next stage is one of consolidation and at this stage the focus is on understanding a particular position and the knowledge and skills that are required, so that the individual can become more confident and competent. The employee may still require support but can be expected to function more independently as he/she clarifies the role and responsibilities and internalises organisational goals, objectives and purpose. Again the length of time in this stage will vary with the position and the individual. Learning activities should vary and could occur both on-the-job and away from the work place. Although the buddy or preceptor may no longer be closely involved, they need to remain available and to continue to take an interest in the employee's progress. This stage is likely to occur over a longer period of time, and may take up to six months. At the completion of this stage, it is useful to conduct an interim review of performance so that learning needs can be identified and goals can be set for future development.

The next stage includes an ongoing process of continuing education, during which the learning centres on the continuing development of attitudes, behaviours and skills to improve performance or may be in response to a change in the position. There is also room for challenge and learning should be future focussed. Activities may be employer or employee initiated and can include inhouse as well as external activities. Learning may be semi-formal as in a workshop, or formal as in the pursuit of a higher qualification, or for either personal or professional growth. It is essential that the organisation recognises the importance of establishing a climate of ongoing learning, seeing growth and development and change as normal, healthy activities.

During a period of employment a promotion may occur which brings the process of staff development back to a period of orientation and consolidation for the new position. Again expectations of performance must be realistic to allow for appropriate preparation for the new position and learning should be planned and not implemented as a crisis measure. Unfortunately, it is often assumed by the employer that with promotion the employee will immediately assume the new position and will not require an orientation or consolidation stage. Little time is made available for settling in to the new position. You can probably think of a person who performed very well in a position, but when promoted, appeared to lose confidence and ability. The phrase, promoted beyond the level of competence, is not uncommon. In many cases this occurs because the individual is not given time to orient to the new position nor given permission to be a learner again.

At some stage of employment, an individual may decide to leave or may be told to leave, which brings the process to the final stage of exit. An employee may retire, resign to take up a new direction, be made redundant, or be dismissed. Regardless of the circumstances the employee wants to finish off the business of the position before leaving. This stage provides an opportunity

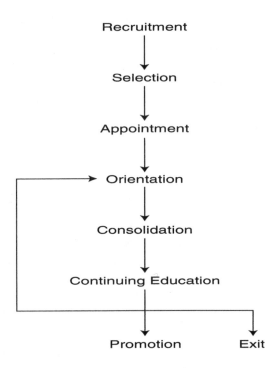

Fig. 1.1 The process of staff development

for the employer to learn a great deal about the position and about the organisation in general. It also provides an opportunity for acknowledgment and recognition of achievement. Feedback to the employe, at the time of an exit interview can be very useful for both parties. Regardless of circumstances, if handled well the separation can be positive.

This process recognises the complexity of staff development. Successful staff development will balance the needs of the organisation with those of the individual, focus activities on need and develop flexible, adaptable strategies using a variety of resources and learning styles. By viewing it as an ongoing process, different strategies which can be implemented at each stag, are linked together and form part of the overall plan.

A framework for planning staff development

Staff development can be viewed from a macro level, meaning overall, and from a micro level, meaning from within. In this way it is placed within a planning framework that addresses both overall purpose and outcomes.

Macro planning

The most important consideration in macro planning is the concept of needs assessment. The purpose of needs assessment is not to suggest solutions but to identify those areas where solutions are most required and to set criteria for their resolution. Needs are questions of values and philosophy and technical methods cannot analyse them completely. Quantitative and qualitative methods are required to take into account all aspects of identified needs. It is important to establish an understanding of the terms need and needs assessment. Three major types of needs have been identified: real needs, educational needs and felt needs.

Types of needs

Real needs:
Deficiencies that exist but may not be recognised by the person
Example: to communicate with staff more effectively.
Educational needs:
Deficiencies in specific skills, attitudes, knowledge that are lacking and which can be met by a learning experience
Example: to learn to communicate assertively rather than aggressively.
Felt needs:
Deficiencies identified and considered important by the individual
Example: to improve self concept and increase self esteem.

The ability to identify needs may be limited by an individual's self awareness and so it is often the role of staff development personnel to assist the individual to recognise and articulate needs.

Needs assessment has been defined by Kaufman (Witkin 1984) as a formal analysis that shows and documents the gaps between current results and desired results (ideally concerned with gaps in outcomes), arranges the gaps (needs) in priority order and selects the needs to be resolved. Witkin (1984) suggests there is some consensus on the definition of a needs assessment but not necessarily on the design. She believes a needs assessment can be a change-oriented process, a method of enumeration, a description of a decision making process. Another way of classifying needs assessment is by the focus on the needs of the individual or the needs of the organisation. Needs assessment is such an integral part of staff development and the design of an appropriate tool is so important that it is discussed in detail in Chapter 2 and therefore will be discussed only briefly here. Needs assessment begins with a number of questions:

- Who wants the assessment?
- Why is the assessment wanted?
- What should be the scope of the assessment?

- On whose needs will it focus?
- What kinds and amounts of data will be collected?
- What methods will be used for data collection?
- What constraints will influence the data collection?

All these questions must be answered as part of the preparation for needs assessment. Needs assessment is not a one-off activity either and if conducted regularly can provide the link between need and outcome. Anyone planning to conduct a needs assessment; that is, a manager or educator, may think he/she knows the staff's needs but this may only be the perception of the manager or educator. Without careful and comprehensive planning needs assessment can become an expensive data collecting activity that produces information of little practical relevance.

Macro planning

Staff development requires the development of a program. Put simply, program development follows several steps:

- identify a need
- establish the goals and set the purpose
- identify the learners and consider their specific characteristics
- define the objectives to reflect the desired outcomes
- identify the preferred learning style
- establish the educational method
- determine the setting
- establish the means of evaluation
- complement the program
- evaluate outcomes against initial needs
- identify needs.

Holland (1987) describes a more complex process, calling it a model for the continuing education process. He believes such a model provides a framework for the rational development of programs and it functions as a guide for marketing as well as production.

Employer–employee relationship

Health care organisations

Debate often occurs over the responsibility for staff development. Is it the employer's responsibility or the employee's responsibility? Should the employee take responsibility for pursuing his/her learning or is it reasonable for the employer to commit resources towards the employee's learning. The most useful solution is to recognise that both employer and employee have a responsibility. The employer should recognise a responsibility to offer

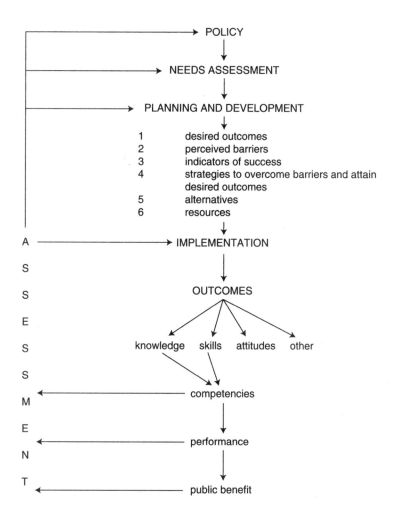

Fig. 1.2 Model for the continuing education process

opportunities for staff development as part of an overall responsibility for the well being of the employee. The employee should recognise a responsibility to keep up to date with the requirements of the job, and accept a professional responsibility to remain competent to practise.

Most people spend many hours at work, establish relationships with colleagues and seek to attain a positive attitude towards their employer. They work to the best of their ability and strive to contribute to the success of the organisation. In return they seek recognition for effort, appropriate financial reward and the opportunity to achieve and to feel they are making a contribution. Staff development is the tool to facilitate a positive relationship between employer and employee and to provide a communication link. The employer can be kept aware of the needs of staff and of the organisational culture and climate, and use this information to anticipate future development of staff. Through staff development, the employee can be provided with the opportunity to hear about organisational plans and goals, be provided with a forum for personal and professional counsel, given an opportunity to get messages to the employer about needs or suggest the direction the organisation might need to take and take advantage of an opportunity to improve performance.

Clearly there is a connection between respect from management for the employee and the enthusiasm the employee displays in the work place. When the employer treats the employee as important, with respect and attention, a significant impact can often be seen in the service that is provided. Health care is a human service, a people business, where the product, health, is hard to define, expensive to attain, and perceived differently by individual members of the client group. It is difficult to develop a normative level of performance or a common expectation for a product or service when you are considering a large and varied client group. Hasenfiled and English in Donovan and Jackson (1991) note a number of distinctive attributes of human service organisations:

- The raw material is human beings all of whom are different.
- Goal definition is problematical and ambiguous.
- Technology is indeterminate.
- Staff-client relationships are the core activities.
- The service relies on professional services.
- The service lacks reliable and valid measures of effectiveness.

For the health care provider, these attributes transform into complexities that make fulfilment of their role more difficult. These complexities are worthy of consideration.

Health care organisations often face multiple conflicting environmental constraints

Sometimes the efforts to respond to one constraint may inhibit the reaction to another. For example, one department may aim to meet client needs in one way, while another department may use a different method. These two different methods, equally appropriate, may not be compatible. Generally, the larger and more complex the organisation the greater the range of constraints and the less likely they can be altered. An uncompromising demand for a quality outcome by an employer, without recognition of the constraints that exist, will do little for staff morale or for the achievement of the outcomes. Staff will make sacrifices if they have had the constraints explained to them. If the employer makes the employee feel as important as the outcomes they desire by using strategies within a staff development program, common realistic goals can be achieved.

Health care organisations often have multiple conflicting goals

An organisation usually has one common goal, sometimes stated as a mission statement or purpose, but individual departments can all have their own goals and purposes. Contradiction between departments over minor goals are a prime source of staff dissatisfaction and can result in activities that act collectively against the attainment of the common goal. Goals can be different providing there is an understanding of the reason for their difference and a climate of co-operation rather than competition between departments. A staff development program based on organisation beliefs and values will ack–nowledge differences but promote common values and outcomes.

Health care organisations have multiple and conflicting external constituents

In this context constituents means people affected by the organisation, such as clients, clients' families and carers, community groups, government, unions, professional organisations and the general community. An expectation of blanket efficiency for all the constituents is not appropriate and signifies an employer who is out of touch with the reality of the environment. A staff development program can ensure that information flows throughout an organisation so that the whole picture is kept in perspective. For example, a hospital may be expected to decrease the budget allocated to after care staff services that it offers, in response to a state government planning policy. The hospital may know, however, that this is a growth area of its business: it will have to increase its budget in this area because the staff working in this area identified in a staff needs assessment survey that they needed education in case planning and clinical home care. The constituents that this hospital is responding to—the government, clients and staff—all had different needs.

The nature of the service is unique and complex

Health care is designed to provide a service geared towards producing a change in the health status of people or the circumstances affecting them. This process is complex and can vary between individuals. Within any client group a range of values will exist which will present as a different response or a different health status. It may be identified that staff need education to assist them to respond appropriately to different values and needs, or to deal with the ethics and complexity of behaviour change associated with health care.

Role of the individual health care provider

The role requires individual strength and often independence and autonomy, yet usually also involves work as part of a team. This diversity calls for particular strengths and expertise. Health care providers are subject to enormous expectations, from within themselves (*I should have done a better job*), from the profession itself (*You should have known how to do that*), and from the community in general (*You should know everything about health care*). Unrealistic expectations are the source of enormous distress and will impact directly on performance. Another factor in this area relates to the very nature of work, that is the things health care providers (nurses, doctors, physio–therapists, chiropractors) do as part of their job. There is often a need to classify work into routine procedures and to remove personal feelings or concerns so that the task can be completed. How many times have you been asked, How can you do all those things? There is an enormous need to recognise the significance of this personal component of health care and to ensure that resources are available for personal as well as professional development. Resources should be provided for debriefing, for learning to manage potential and actual stressful situations, for time out or relocation to another area, or for counselling in response to particular situations. All these activities are important human resource activities and should all fall within the responsibilities of a comprehensive staff development function.

Partnership between employer and employee

Research into the needs of the staff within a large health care organisation in Western Australia (Horner 1990) identified the following employee needs:

- congruence with the values of the organisation
- job satisfaction in two dimensions: first, from the relationship with clients, and second, from the relationship with the employer
- satisfactory work environment incorporating such things as privacy, adequate resources, personal space and safe work conditions
- recognisable career pathway with opportunities for advancement
- confidence in the leader or manager
- personal feelings of worth.

These needs form the basis of a good quality work life, which has been defined by Mirvis and Lawler (1984) as one that attracts employees, trains and develops them, advances them with enriching work experiences, invites their participation in job related and organisational decisions and, at the same time, provides them with a stable environment, adequate income and benefits and a secure place to work. With a quality work life, the employee is likely to make a commitment to the organisation, its values and beliefs, and will work to attain quality outcomes. In reality, people's needs are not complex.

People's work related needs

- To feel valued and have their efforts recognised and rewarded
- To have an active role in the management of the organisation
- To feel some sense of responsibility for the outcomes of the organisation
- To see opportunities for growth and development, and to feel challenged

Mutual commitment results in a partnership between employer and employee and can be achieved through the following strategies:

- commitment to employees through a staff development program
- recognition and acknowledgment of performance through regular constructrve formal and informal feedback
- regular, employer-initiated demonstration that employees are valued
- open honest communication which recognises the input of all parties
- effective management of change that involves all those affected.

Many management strategies and styles are in existence today in health care organisations. Common terms for strategies include decentralisation, regionalisation, flat management structures, total quality management, shared governance, and you have probably heard many more. Some of these strategies will be explored in Chapter 5 when the process of staff development is examined in more detail as part of management practices. Regardless of the theory or the term that is current at the time, the most important and most significant factor is the relationship that is created between employer and employee. That is what makes the difference.

Chapter summary

Staff development in the work place should be no longer an option. Maximum performance cannot be achieved, nor productivity realised without a commitment to staff development. Health care today demands excellence in performance and a high quality of service, where service refers to the care that is being delivered. Such high standards can be achieved only if the human resources, that is the staff of the organisation, are considered as important as either the physical or financial resources. This chapter has looked at the meaning of staff development in terms of an eight-stage process of staff development, where a strong relationship is established between employer and employee. Terms that are important to the understanding of staff development have been described, such as quality of work life and human resource management. Finally, this chapter has presented both a framework for staff development in terms of planning and an explanation of how the partnership between employer and employee can be developed to facilitate growth and development and a commitment to long term learning.

REFERENCES

Brennan B (ed) 1990 Continuing professional education, promise and performance. ACER, Radford House, Victoria

Donovan F, Jackson A C 1991 Managing human service organisations. Prentice Hall, Sydney

Gathers B J 1988 Issues in mandatory staff development. Journal of Nursing Staff Development 120-124

Holland R W 1987 A theoretical framework for the process of CPE. In: Dymock D R (ed) Continuing Education Conference, University of New England, Oct 36-48

Horner B 1990 Needs assessment for staff development in the Silver Chain Nursing Association. University of Western Australia Press, Perth

Horsefield G 1988 Managing the human asset in the public sector. Peat Marwick Hungerfords Management Consultants, Melbourne

Levine M F 1983 Self development QWL measures. Journal of Occupational Behaviour 4:35-46

Mirvis P H, Lawler E 1983 Accounting for the quality of work life. Journal of Occupational Behaviour A5: 197-212

Witkin B R 1984 Assessing needs in education and social programs. Jossy Bass Publishers, San Francisco

2

Needs assessment

Key questions

- What part does needs assessment play in staff development?
- What needs assessment instruments are effective?
- How would you develop a needs assessment questionnaire?
- How can you develop a staff development program from needs?
- What are common areas of need in staff development?

Content summary

Introduction

Needs assessment

    Needs

    Information obtained from needs assessment

        Information obtained from a needs assessment

        Management information

        Individual staff information

Needs assessment in health care

    A three-way partnership

    Categories of individual need (staff needs)

        Needs commonly identified by staff

Needs assessment instruments

    Interview

    Questionnaire

    Observation

    Workshops

Developing a needs assessment instrument

Program planning based on need

    Employee learning needs

    Quality of work life factors

    General and psychological health

Common areas of need

    Update of clinical expertise

    Workload management

    Occupational stress

References

Introduction

Needs assessment is an integral part of planning for staff development. It does not end with the collection and analysis of data but extends into the program planning phase, guiding the selection of solutions to staff development needs.

Changing needs in education for health care professions where obsolescence and technical advancement are a daily reality, has been affirmed by individuals and organisations. What are staff needs? How can we obtain this information and how can we use it? What benefits can be identified? How much will it cost? These questions are often asked by individuals charged with res-ponsibilities in staff development.

In terms of job skills and performance, needs assessment is an effort to reveal the gap between what people do at work and what the employer would like them to do, that is, the process of validating the discrepancies between current levels of output and those the system hopes to attain.

This chapter discusses needs assessment in terms of process and method for staff development in health care; describes the most common types of needs assessment instruments; explains how to develop a useful instrument; relates needs assessment to the development of a program; and presents the most commonly identified staff needs.

Needs assessment

An essential component of planning in staff development is a systematic, relatively objective way of assessing needs in order to make decisions about priorities for services or programs. The purpose of needs assessment is not to make decisions about priorities, but to identify those areas where solutions are most required and to set criteria for their solution.

Needs

Needs have been described in many different ways. They are a question of value and philosophy and require a comprehensive methodology and analysis using both quantitative and qualitative methods to take into account all aspects of identified needs. Needs can be assessed at different levels. Moroney in Witkin (1984) has identified four categories of needs in human services:

- normative needs: services that are needed for a client population, for example, transport for day surgery clients
- perceived needs: what individuals consider their needs to be, for example, the need for acceptance and understanding
- expressed needs: revealed by the individual, for example, policies on the legal liability of staff when clients go home less than 24 hours after surgery
- relative needs: a gap in existing services/knowledge/expertise, for example, a clinical procedure relative to a new surgical technique.

Kristjanson and Scanlan (1989) describe need in terms of staff development as *educational* needs and *felt* needs. An *educational* need results from an educational deficiency, implying an attempt to attain a goal (e.g. to be able to manage work load more effectively) and which can be met by a learning activity (a session on developing tools to assess work load and plan activities into a series of steps). A *felt* need is one considered important by the individual (e.g. to write documentation objectively) but which may not be perceived to be important to anyone else. A felt need is often limited by the individual's self awareness: are they aware that there is a gap in their performance or have a desire to improve performance?

Another way to categorise needs has been suggested by Beach (1984) who explains needs within a four part framework that he calls a Johari Window (where each part represents a pane of the window). He categorises needs in this way:

- blind needs: staff may be unaware of a need but management may have identified this need through audits or records or appraisal
- shared needs: staff and management may have identified the same need through a survey tool or records, audits or appraisal
- hidden needs: staff may identify a need which is unknown by management
- undiscovered needs: needs that result from changes to work practices that have not yet been recognised through records, audits or appraisal.

There is some value in defining the type of need, as in the discussion above, if it helps to categorise the source or assists the development of a plan for action. But it is far more important to recognise the purpose of identifying needs. Needs assessment is a change oriented process, a method for enumeration and description or a decision making process.

Providing the person conducting the assessment describes how they are using the term and the purpose of the exercise, that is, what they intend to do with the information they discover, the classification can remain secondary. Needs assessment is not useful if it is an academic/management exercise that takes up a lot of time and has no measurable, visible outcome.

Information obtained from needs assessment

Needs assessment for staff development usually refers to educational needs. When properly conducted, needs assessment can provide information about different types of needs, all of which can be critical to the success of any staff development program designed to address gaps in performance.

This volume of information can only be obtained if *all parties* are involved and committed to the activity; that is, if everyone recognises that everyone's needs are important. It is important to include staff working in positions, subject matter experts, managers, clients, and people who have held the position and moved on. All categories of staff are important as they all have valuable information and opinions to contribute and the cumulative knowledge they supply reflects a variety of perspectives.

Information obtained from a needs assessment

- Scope: the content covered, what topics should and should not be included
- Theme: the relationship to a position, why an employee should participate
- Central topics/key issues: teaching areas which can be based on performance objectives
- Most common procedures: the activities most often associated with a job or process
- Most common duties, tasks and steps: specific job responsibilities for an individual
- Efficiency concerns: factors affecting overall performance
- Alternative approaches to performance: processes and procedures that work but are not found in standard documentation
- Service expectations: issues deemed important by users of the service
- Perceived importance of topics: standardised ratings of topics
- Perceived levels of knowledge/skill: self appraisals of present levels
- Learning preference: preferred methods for giving and receiving information
- Links to other staff development: the relationship between current performance, prerequisites or advanced levels
- Risks analysis: estimated losses or costs to the organisation if a program is cancelled or delayed
- Side issues: nice-to-know information picked up along the way

Information from needs assessment might be useful to management and/or individual staff:

Management information

- evaluation of present performance
- identification of factors influencing cost effectiveness
- measure of the outcomes of past activities
- awareness of unmet current needs

Individual staff information

- awareness of management's commitment
- feedback on performance and service delivery
- clarification of roles and responsibilities
- identification of skill and knowledge deficits.

The list of possible uses of the information from a needs assessment is endless, limited only by the individuals conducting the assessment and the creativity and flexibility of the work environment.

Needs assessment in health care

A three-way partnership

Needs assessment in health care involves a three-way partnership between the service provider (the staff development provider), the service receiver (the staff) and the stakeholders (the employer and the client). Each partner benefits from needs assessment in slightly different ways.

For the *service provider*, needs assessment benefits program planning and evaluation. It identifies and ranks needs while examining the effectiveness and worth of existing programs/services in relation to the needs that have been identified. Needs assessment tends to address future oriented questions (What should we be pursuing; where should we be heading?), as well as past oriented questions (What have we achieved; how successful have we been?).

Application

Staff state in a needs assessment questionnaire that the characteristics of the client population have changed as a result of earlier discharge practices. They state that they need education on client education strategies to ensure that clients go home well informed about their progress and alert to any changes in condition. This information tells the service provider the focus and content of a session that should be planned for staff.

The *service receiver* gains by the identification of learning needs that relate to their job environment, their work practices and/or the level of job satisfaction. They value their work more as their needs are being met.

Application

Staff feel they do not have the skills and knowledge to present a good teaching session to clients in the shortened time that is available to them, because they will be going home several days earlier than has been past practice. Their needs are identified and met through a teaching session. This results in the development of a pictorial chart that shows all that the client needs to know, accompanied by a brochure explaining the chart that the clients take home with them. The teaching can be done in minimal time and the knowledge can be reinforced by the brochure.

The *stakeholders* also both gain and their benefits are closely linked. The employer gains because feedback from clients indicates satisfaction with the service; the clients gain because they receive a good service and have received value for money in terms of their care.

Application

The employer notices the quality of the material that is going home with the client. From feedback sheets clients are asked to complete on Quality of Service she sees how well received the material is by the client. Satisfied clients will return and will speak positively to other people, so business is assured. Staff are working effectively and are satisfied and so might be expected to stay in the job and those responsible for staff development are achieving outcomes that are measurable.

This may seem a simplistic explanation where everyone lives happily ever after. However, the inter-relationship does not have to be complex to be valuable. What does show is that the identification of one need or set of needs, that is, strategies for client education in response to earlier discharge practices, which is addressed within a staff development strategy, can bring results to all partners. The ultimate goal is cost effective, quality client care within the existing health care system, delivered by competent staff who feel they are doing a good job and meeting their clients needs. This is assisted by informed, relevant staff development. What more could anyone want?

Categories of individual need (staff needs)

Within the three-way partnership, it is the needs of the staff that are most relevant to this discussion, so their needs will be looked at in more detail. Individuals' needs can be generalised to some extent. Hunt (1986) refers to eight recurring categories of need, which he calls goal categories, in his book on managing people at work. I refer to his goals as *needs* because they align with what I have identified in my research.

Needs commonly identified by staff

1 The need for comfort
2 The need for structure
3 The need for relationships
4 The need for recognition and status
5 The need for power
6 The need for autonomy
7 The need for creativity
8 The need for growth

Hunt claims that although the broad category of a need may remain relatively stable there are subtle shifts of emphasis within the need. Needs are not static. They shift over time within individuals and between individuals in the work place. The precise content of needs and the order in which they might be ranked is, of course, subject to individual perception and may change. An examination of these categories can provide a useful framework for staff development.

The need for comfort

These needs may be referred to as a body of primary needs and include food, drink and shelter, but in the work environment they refer to the physiological comfort of pleasant working conditions, the minimisation of distress caused by work related pressures or (unrealistic) expectations and satisfactory reward or remuneration. These needs can be summarised as those needs that result in a comfortable work lifestyle. There is considerable variability within this category based upon social and economic background and personal motiv- ational forces.

Many employees will rate comfort goals as a low priority in relation to other goals as they fully expect them to be met. It is often presumed that health professionals are not interested or concerned about salary as they see their work as a calling or not of monetary value. The salary may not be what attracts people to a job, but if it is perceived that they are not being paid what they believe they are worth, or there is obvious disparity between groups, salary can be the source of considerable job dissatisfaction. No-one likes to be taken advantage of nor to feel devalued in comparison with another equally qualified and experienced practitioner. Comfort needs may not be as important as others, but if the basics are not in place, it is difficult to move beyond that point. For example, it is unreasonable to expect staff to perform at full potential if the ward facilities are sub-standard, the equipment malfunctions or the salary rates are under award. It is important to ensure basic needs are met first.

The need for structure

Structure, certainty and security needs are closely linked to comfort needs and the two sets are often difficult to separate. Organisations have traditionally relied on structure and threats of insecurity to control behaviour of employees. If employees deviated from the required behaviour patterns they were threatened with the sack (and insecurity), isolation (and insecurity) or promotional restrictions (failure and insecurity). Structure based on control and discipline is often based on insecurity even if the outcome is presented as necessary and a means of self control.

Structure, certainty and security are significant in some positions and for some individuals. If these are high level needs, the individual will probably find difficulty dealing with rapidly changing environments and conditions. If they like routine and doing the same thing in the same way, with little creativity or variability, they may identify needs in terms of, *If only things would just stabilise for a while and we could get used to doing things the same way,* or *I can't stand all this change, why can't we go back to the good old days.* Have you heard these statements before? In health care, for example in nursing, many procedures need to remain the same because that is how we know the standard will be maintained and the care consistent. People develop habits and become used to doing things the same way and, if structure, certainty and security is important to them, they will react against changes to methods and/or procedures. Changes to nursing education from hospital-based programs to tertiary-based programs and the reactions of nurses, doctors, other health professionals and the public in some cases, is an excellent example of where needs for structure, certainty and security can still be challenged.

The need for relationships

Individuals with strong relationship needs will seek out employment situations where they can form lasting relationships. These employment situations are often identified to be a characteristic of the caring professions, such as the health care professions. Hunt (1986) claims that approximately 60% of the work force will identify relationship needs as their highest level of need, not advancement or achievement at work. Health care work involves the establishment of relationships with colleagues and clients, and this activity can make a significant difference to what is perceived to be a good outcome in any interaction. It is unlikely that you would stay in health care if you were a person who did not feel comfortable interacting and talking with people. Relationships with colleagues and managers can make a significant difference to how we work and to the level of job satisfaction we attain. Needs in this area may be less visible than clinical skills or a knowledge deficit, but they are particularly important.

The need for recognition and status

Studies on motivation often links these needs together, but it is useful to see them as two sets of needs. First, needs which reflect a desire for recognition from others and second, needs which reflect a desire to manage and control the activities of others. The importance of recognition as a need is that it provides employers and managers with opportunities to reward behaviour and achievement. On the other hand, it can be an enormous source of dissatisfaction if employees feel their efforts are unrecognised. Status needs relate to an individual's desire for promotion, sometimes described as career aspirations. Individuals who rate status needs as important usually seek opportunities to demonstrate their expertise and will often pursue promotional positions and/ or formal further education and qualifications.

The need for power

A power need relates to a need to influence, control and reward behaviour. For many managers it is this need that rates more strongly than that of recognition or status. One of the difficulties of separating a power need from a recognition need is that employers may mix power and status together and so reinforce the authority of the position rather than the characteristics of the person. This results in what are perceived to be perks of a position and does not necessarily relate to ability or performance. There is always the potential for this category of need to turn into self need at the expense of another and it is worth analysing the many other needs of an individual or group before responding to this need alone.

The need for autonomy, creativity and growth

Hunt considers these three needs as dependent upon each other and so considers them together. In terms of need, theorists write about the concept of self-actualisation or self-fulfilment as being the ultimate or end point of development. Both are extremely difficult to measure and for many individuals they are never attained because their needs continue to change as they aspire to reach this ultimate state. Many individuals who seek autonomy also seek creativity, whether they recognise this or not. However, a need for autonomy and/or creativity will usually result in growth. Autonomy can be described as a search for independence rather than dependence, for control of oneself rather than control of others. Opportunities for originality and creativity may exist within a need for autonomy, but both may not always be found in the same person. Finally, a search for growth and challenge, extending the boundaries and stretching for options, often demonstrates as a need for autonomy. In essence, the need for both autonomy and creativity result in growth.

In summary, all these categories of need can be seen within an organisation and within an individual. When needs are identified, it is always important to view needs as part of a total picture as few needs are isolated. A thorough needs assessment can identify a great deal of useful information about individuals in their work setting. It is important to remember that an individual's personal needs will often be represented within a work need and the influence of one upon another should be recognised.

Needs assessment instruments

Needs assessment can be as simple as asking someone what programs they would like to attend or as complex as a multiple question survey for computerised factor analysis. The purpose of the assessment will often guide the choice of instrument. The steps in the design of an instrument will be discussed with reference to a questionnaire, one of the most common instruments. Other common instruments are the interview, observation and workshops. A thorough needs assessment should include more than one instrument at any one time, to develop a comprehensive staff development program. All methods have their uses and all will suit the situation, the individual and the outcome, at different times. It is valuable to experiment with them all over time and to work out how you can best use them.

Interview

An interview can vary from very structured (specific questions with answers categorised and coded) to very unstructured (*tell me about* questions). A great deal of the variation will depend on the time and resources available to the interviewer as well as on the purpose of the interview. Questions can be closed, seeking yes/no answers or quite specific details, or open, seeking individual interpretation of the information that is required. Interviews can be standardised so that they are the same for each individual or can remain quite unstructured.

A standardised interview has these characteristics:

* aims to obtain a set of views from a number of individuals
* asks items in a set order
* all questions are pre-tested in a pilot study
* results can be codified
* suits homogenous groups and large numbers.

An unstructured interview has these characteristics:

* aims to get an insight into an issue using open questions
* there are no set items; rather people are encouraged to talk
* practice is required to identify the key/important points
* suits heterogenous groups, few numbers and requires considerable time.

Questionnaire

Questionnaires or surveys are a common method of obtaining information. The fact that a large number of respondents can be reached with the same tool is often seen to be a significant advantage of this instrument. If the questionnaire is mailed out or sent out to individuals and no opportunity exists to supervise its completion, both the number and quality of returns can influence the usefulness of the information. A follow up strategy is advisable to increase the validity of the data. Questionnaires can, however, be very useful if the purpose is clearly identified.

Questionnaires can be designed to elicit a variety of information in that different types of questions can be asked. The advantage of anonymity should not be overlooked either. A considerable amount of data can be obtained from a questionnaire, which when analysed can effectively identify specific needs. Questionnaires are very useful in the identification of topics or specific skills, where the participant is given a series of topics or skills to choose from, or to place in priority order. Questionnaires can include open and closed questions and can also elicit qualitative data. The data from a questionnaire can be coded and analysed readily and this computerised method of data analysis can bring meaning to a large quantity and variety of information.

Observation

Observation can be a very effective instrument if well planned but requires careful consideration to avoid feelings of intimidation by those being observed. The observer needs to identify clearly what it is they wish to look for, behaviours, lack of behaviours, specific activities, verbal and/or non-verbal communication, the existence or absence of skills, and so on. The observer requires astute powers of observation and the ability to remain in focus and not be distracted by extraneous events.

Usually the information is collected unedited and then a long and laborious effort is put into analysing, coding and making sense of the data. It is a time consuming and therefore a costly method of obtaining information. A great deal of skill is needed in managing the observation, asking questions, clarifying observations, verifying data and then, finally, the analysis is usually given back to the subject for further verification and comment. Few staff development departments would have the resources to use this type of needs assessment instrument. However, in a small department or with a small number of staff, a great deal can be learned by simply observing behaviour that is occurring in the normal course of a day. As an informal tool for collecting data, that is, spending time in an area observing and taking note of behaviours and activities, it can be extremely revealing.

Workshops

Workshops provide an opportunity for the use of a number of different strategies in the same setting. A workshop brings people together for a common purpose and with careful facilitation and a supportive environment, much information can be obtained.

Workshop means, by definition, that participants and facilitator *work*, but because people with similar interests and work experiences are brought together they assist each other to participate. A workshop may start out with a specific purpose, but because people are given the opportunity to mix and share, it is sometimes a challenge to keep it on track. On the other hand, you may consciously decide to let it go in its own direction and to gather the information at the end.

The activities within the workshop become the crucial part of the data collection process. Individuals at work often really enjoy an opportunity to get together with colleagues, in work time, and will grasp this chance to identify needs and talk about work practices enthusiastically. Providing the structures are in place, they can be the most rewarding method of needs assessment. Activities you might use in a workshop include:

- working in pairs on a topic or to answer questions; working with a partner can be less threatening than the whole group.
- feedback to the whole group with someone recording information on a white board or paper; if someone else says it others will often add their opinion.

- small group exercises where the participants work on problems or solutions; common areas of interest and need can be identified.
- games and exercises that create unity and establish supports during the course of the workshop and into the work environment later; exercises are planned with a purpose in mind but appear as a game.
- team activities where individuals work on similar needs to solve problems and identify solutions; individuals gain confidence when someone else appears to think as they do.

The work in preparing, the energy to implement and the work of making sense out of the results can be time consuming and quite exhausting, but the quality of the information can make all this worthwhile. It is useful to have more than one person involved with the running of the workshop, to share the load and bounce off ideas. Clearly, the greater the variety and creativity, the greater the results.

Developing a needs assessment instrument

Regardless of the instrument of choice, there are a series of stages in the development of a needs assessment instrument. In this illustration I have used a questionnaire as the example because it continues to be the instrument used most. The questionnaire is being developed to conduct a needs assessment in a large community-based health care organisation.

There are five main stages in developing the instrument as outlined below:

Stage one: an analysis of the specific context, aims and objectives of the needs assessment

The context originates from the belief that organisational effectiveness will improve with maximum utilisation of the employees' talents and skills which will develop when the employees perceive they have a good quality of working life. The attainment of quality of working life balances the needs of the individual with the needs of the organisation.

The aim is to determine the discrepancy between the existing and needed competencies of staff. It must recognise the significance of the three-way partnership between service provider (staff development department), service receivers (the staff) and the stakeholders (health care organisation and clients). Staff who share a common commitment with the organisation to deliver high quality client care based on client needs are more likely to work towards the attainment of that goal if they perceive the organisation values them and their efforts.

The objectives of the assessment are to identify educational needs in three main categories: job-related skills (what they do), job-related knowledge (what they need to know), and personal and professional development (interpersonal and professional needs and advancement). The assessment also aims to identify those factors perceived to be important to staff in the areas of job satisfaction, working environment, career opportunities and health in the work place, all of which are important for a quality work life.

Stage two: the development of a conceptual framework in light of the context, aims and objectives

The conceptual framework is important for two reasons. First, to ensure the instrument is logical and that it covers the areas of interest systematically in terms of the items and the way the questions are asked. Second, there are implications for the analysis of the data based on the conceptual framework, particularly at the data reduction stage of analysis. The conceptual framework gives structure to both the questionnaire and to the analysis of its data.

The conceptual framework proceeds from answers to questions such as, What exactly is the investigation trying to find out? It should specify the general factors or variables and the specific dimensions or aspects of those factors, so defining the information sought. The conceptual framework will guide the structure and items within questions. In the questionnaire used as an example, the conceptual framework consisted of four sections:

Conceptual framework for a questionnaire

Identification of employees' learning needs:
job-related knowledge
job-related skills
personal/professional education
Identification of quality of work life factors:
feelings towards the employer
relationship with the employer
career pathways
leadership patterns
job satisfaction
Identification of general and psychological health:
a multi-faceted series of questions
Demographic details:
position in the organisation
work classification
length of employment
employment qualifications

Stage three: the generation of measures: items, subscales and scales to flesh out the questionnaire

Certain questions can assist with the development at this stage.

Will I use my own measures or those already in the literature?
The potential for greater validity lies in developing your own measures and you can tailor questions and items to the purpose of the assessment. But established measures will have already established reliability that can be important in multiple item questions, common to this kind of instrument. For example, if I ask this question this way (my way) can I be reasonably sure (statistically and empirically) that the answer is reliable and valid, or could the question be interpreted in another way or the answer mean something else? Good scales are not easy to develop and so it is advisable, certainly in the early days, to use something that has been established and proven.

Do I want to classify responses or scale them?
Data can be classified as *nominal* or *continuous*. Examples of nominal data include sex, country of origin, position in an organisation and qualifications. Data can be classified as *continuous* and used for scaling respondents. Examples of continuous data include socio-economic status, level of commitment, attitude and health status. The statistical significance of distinguishing the nature of the data relates to how it is analysed; that is, different analysis is used for nominal data than for continuous data and they should not be mixed. Strictly speaking, nominal data should be analysed using techniques such as chi square or contingency coefficients, whereas continuous data should be analysed using more powerful techniques such as correlation and regression analysis or analysis of variance.

This may not seem relevant to you, or it may have introduced language and principles not familiar to you at this stage. It is important, however, to understand that the collection of the data in needs assessment is not haphazard and should be planned and executed carefully for the results to be meaningful, reliable and valid. You may need to seek assistance in the design and again at the analysis stage and this is readily available. But you will be asked the same questions; that is, what is the purpose of the assessment and what do you want to measure. By introducing the terminology at the planning stage, your instrument will be well thought out.

What scaling technique do I want to use?
Scaling relates to the measurement of variables and there are three main techniques. The first two are less well known, *equal appearing* (Thurstone) and *cumulative* (Guttman) and I will not explain them here, because the third technique is far more common and is frequently used in questionnaire design. The third technique is a *summative* technique (Likert scale).

The Likert scale has become popular especially in the social science area. Again, there are considerations at this stage of development. Questionnaire scales or sub-scales should measure only one thing, a principle called *uni-dimensionality*. If this is related back to the conceptual framework, it means that variables must be defined in uni-dimensional terms even if it means more sub-divisions to the variable. For example, *employees' feelings about their employer* is a general variable and is multi-dimensional, so this variable needs to be defined in terms of sub-variables such as support for the organisation's philosophy, perceptions of the work environment and potential for career advancement.

So the questionnaire includes those sub-questions, which measure only one thing within that main question, which measures many things. At the analysis stage, uni-dimensional analysis is measured by techniques like inter-item correlation analysis and factor analysis.

A question aims to produce variability among respondents to obtain a good cross section of information represented within response categories for a question. The Likert format suggests more rather than fewer response categories. The most common Likert response format is an agreement scale to each item ranging from *strongly agree to strongly disagree*. It is advisable to use either four or six categories. Studies have shown that a middle or neutral category is inappropriate as the respondent often selects this category if they don't understand the question or can't make up their mind. This does not present useful data (see Table 2.1).

Table 2.1 Question using a Likert scale

For each statement below circle the number on the scale of 1-6 that best describes your feelings about people.

Strong agreement	SA	1
Moderate agreement	MA	2
Agreement	A	3
Disagreement	D	4
Moderate disagreement	MD	5
Strong disagreement	SD	6

	SA	MA	A	D	MD	SD
Client needs always come first	1	2	3	4	5	6
Everyone has the right to maximise their potential	1	2	3	4	5	6
Individual privacy should be respected	1	2	3	4	5	6
All people are basically good	1	2	3	4	5	6
Most people care about others	1	2	3	4	5	6

Individual items are generated for all questions for the specific needs assessment and principles of good writing, grammar and clear meaning all apply. This is time consuming but will make the difference to the number and quality of responses.

Stage four: informal pretest of the questionnaire

It is important to trial the questionnaire before final printing. Usually a small sample of typical respondents is used and they are asked to comment on:

- misunderstanding within questions
- ambiguities of meaning
- possible items that have been missed
- procedural aspects for dissemination.

It is best if the trial can be conducted in small groups with respondents willing to discuss all items of the questionnaire. At this stage, you are not interested in their responses to questions but rather in any misunderstanding or difficulty in responding. Be prepared for questions and misunderstandings and see all comments as a way to increase the validity and reliability of the results rather than as a criticism of your ability. Sometimes something as simple as the way questions are ordered and how they are placed on the paper can significantly influence a response rate. It is far better to find this out at the pretest stage.

The individuals who are involved in the pretest may be able to assist you to disseminate the questionnaire and to act as support for respondents. They can add a measure of credibility to the exercise by verifying the value and usefulness of the assessment.

Stage five: finalisation and implementation

Feedback is incorporated from stage four and the questionnaire should now be finalised. In both the presentation of the final questionnaire and in the procedures used for its administration the intention should be to maximise both the response rate and the validity of responses. Apart from attending to the visual impression and the professional nature of the instrument, a covering letter should be developed to explain the reason for the assessment, to enlist co-operation and to reveal the purpose of the assessment. A word or two from management or the employer always adds a measure of credibility. Con-fidentiality and anonymity should be guaranteed, although in many cases individuals will identify themselves and often reveal a great deal of information not actually requested in the assessment. For some individuals the opportunity to talk to someone may be too important to ignore. Contact details are essential and should be included in the covering letter and perhaps also within the questionnaire. Envelopes need to be provided for returned questionnaires and a central place for collection.

If it is possible, provide opportunities for individuals to answer the questionnaire in work time and to provide a room where someone can be available to answer questions while it is completed. It may also be useful to follow up after a period of time with a reminder letter or memo reminding people of the deadline for return and it may be necessary to utilise more specific or direct measures if the response rate is not satisfactory.

In summary, the design of a good instrument requires considerable effort. There are many things that can influence its success. Any instrument needs careful planning as a badly designed instrument not only fails at that time, but can negatively affect future attempts.

Program planning based on need

The questionnaire used as an example here aimed to identify staff development needs in four areas (see the section on conceptual framework). The findings discussed demonstrate how the needs that were identified would become the foundation of a staff development program. The organisation involved was a large community based health care organisation which provided nursing, personal, and home care to clients in their homes by a staff of roughly 2000 (Horner 1991).

Employee learning needs

Job-related knowledge

Needs were identified in the clinical role and in other areas. Staff were asked to rate thirty items classified as job - related knowledge. The topics which were identified by a 50% or greater response rate in this research were considered significant. The topics were:

- loss and grief
- coping with death and dying
- working with people with disabilities
- communication
- basic life support techniques
- pain management
- infection control
- behaviour change in illness
- specific client conditions: further opportunities were given to identify specific topics.

Job-related skills

Staff were asked to rate 27 items classified as job-related skills. Again, the topics identified by a 50% or greater response rate were considered significant. The topics were:

- lifting and transferring clients
- dealing with difficult clients
- listening skills
- thinking logically
- caring for client's physical needs in the home
- clinical nursing skills: further opportunities were given to identify specific topics.

Personal and professional education

Staff were asked to rate 32 items classified as personal or professional education. The topics identified by a 50% or greater response rate were considered significant. The topics were:

- community resources for clients
- effective communication
- basic first aid.

Topics identified by just less than a 50% response rate were also considered significant and these topics were:

- learning to relax
- healthy lifestyle behaviour
- awareness of personal health
- managing stress at work.

These results were organisation wide and formed the foundation of a program. Individual department results allowed for more specific planning. Other information was obtained from other questions (figures rounded to nearest whole number).

Other information

Preferred format:

one-day seminar	36%
half-day seminar	32%
short session	17%
self-directed packages	17%

Preferred time:

morning	47%
afternoon	29%
evening	8%
week-end	6%

Preferred style:

workshop	48%
lecture/talk	19%
tutorial/discussion	15%
video	6%
case study	5%
audio	2%

From these results it can be seen that it would not be cost effective to invest resources into the production of video tapes. Neither would it be effective to run programs on weekends nor to develop self-directed learning packages.

Quality of work life factors

Respondents strongly agreed with the organisation's motto (73%) and name (92%), as presenting an accurate image of the organisation. This was reinforced with comments on the philosophy of the organisation. It could be surmised from these results that there was not a need to build commitment to the organisation or to address issues of employer-employee conflict.

Respondents were positive about the working environment rating highly such items as privacy, noise levels, appropriate equipment, adequate resources, amenities, personal space and safe working conditions. Respondents were less positive about career pathways. Forty-four indicated that they were not encouraged to advance their career nor had they received information about opportunities, of which there were very few. Topics on career information and career counselling might thus be included in a staff development program.

Items relating to perceptions of managers and leaders identified a number of interesting issues. Many respondents stated they were reluctant to answer or had difficulty understanding this section, not a surprising situation as employees often feel reluctant to express honest feelings about managers or bosses. Issues of delegation without control, lack of consultation on decisions, presence or absence of feedback on performance and honest open communication were all revealed. The quantity and type of information from this section indicated that further examination of these topics should be pursued and that the needs identified warranted careful consideration and action by the researcher.

Job satisfaction from an employer-employee perspective did not rate higher than a moderate level. However, job satisfaction from an employee-client perspective rated far more highly. This is not uncommon in health care where relationships with clients is considered very important. Two issues arise from these needs. First, the employer should realise that they don't rate highly and second, the importance of the client should not be underestimated.

General and psychological health

In this section a frequently used and well validated instrument was incorporated into the questionnaire for this section, Goldberg's General Health Ques–tionnaire: GHQ (Van Schoubroeck 1986). Normative data is available from large samples of the Australian population. The analysis of the data, collected from a series of statements rated 1-4, is collapsed into two numbers. They are added together to get a total score for an individual, with a score of 5 or more indicating levels of tension, anxiety or depression, perhaps high enough to affect the individual's health or well being. The total score between 0 and 5 indicates a LOW level of tension, a total score between 5 and 10 indicates a MEDIUM level of tension, and a total score between 10 and 30 indicates a HIGH level of tension.

Overall results did not present findings of concern but some scores within individual departments warranted closer consideration. Distress in the work place can arise from a number of factors:

- relationships with clients
- relationships with colleagues
- physical/environmental factors
- conflict or difficulty with the role
- unrealistic expectations of performance
- insecurity
- lack of guidelines/policies.

If results had indicated high levels of tension there would have been a need to look for sources of tension and perhaps to look at programs on stress awareness, relaxation techniques, balancing work and personal life, assertive behaviour, self concept and/or communication techniques.

Any needs assessment will provide opportunities for staff to comment on issues other than those included within the instrument. Some of the other comments will be positive and may provide useful information, for example, *This is the first time I have felt I could express my opinion.* Other comments will be negative or even angry, for example, *I resent having these personal questions asked of me,* and *No wonder we are broke and can't provide services when you are wasting money on this sort of thing.* It is important to accept all comments as another source of information and to learn from them as much as you can.

Finally, it can be seen from this summary of the results that a great deal of information was obtained from the needs assessment, much of which could be used in program planning. If further understanding is needed, it may be necessary to reduce or analyse information or to use another method for clarification, for example, interviews or workshops.

Common areas of need

There is often an expectation held by health care organisations that the nature of the business as human and caring will be demonstrated within the management of the human resources. In other words, because the business is about meeting clients' needs, management will be good at identifying staff needs. This, of course, is not necessarily the case. Staff need to be viewed as another category of client equally as important as the client who receives the service, perhaps even more so. Staff needs are often lost (referred to as the forgotten client) within the organisation's needs and/or those of the client, both of which appear more visible.

Staff needs can be as variable as the individuals themselves. Fortunately, the literature now recognises some common themes of need in health care organisations based on the nature of the service. The three common themes are:

- update of clinical expertise
- work load management
- occupational stress.

The intention of identifying these three themes is not to pre-empt needs but rather to alert you to common themes, and perhaps to help you make sense of a difficult and diverse area.

Update of clinical expertise

Skill development and skill transfer are particularly important aspects of staff development. They demand accurate knowledge of the skills required, the skills performed and the actual level of skill among employees. Simply put, this means knowing what skills are needed, how to do them, and how well they are being done. It is often difficult to standardise skills and equally as difficult to assess them. There is a need for personal experience and credibility among those staff making any sort of judgement. It is often a challenge to stimulate staff to keep up to date by allowing them to develop expertise for new areas of practice in anticipation of new demand, while ensuring that they maintain the expertise needed for the current situation.

There is also a challenge at the management level. There is not only a need for staff development for current managers and managers-in-training but also a requirement to anticipate needs for future managers. Managers of the future may also have different expertise and experience and may present different needs. Managers within health care in the future may not have the traditional expertise and experience of the discipline in which they work. There is considerable debate about whether managers in health care should be expert in their profession before they become managers, or whether the need is for a good manager regardless of professional clinical expertise. This situation will present a challenge for the staff development provider who may have a wider client group to work with.

Another issue in management relates to the situation where an excellent clinician is promoted to a management position and fails hopelessly. It has been assumed that because the person was eligible for promotion they will automatically handle the new position. Their specific needs have not been identified.

Workload management

People often say, *I need to learn to manage my time better.* The truth is, you cannot manage time for it just keeps ticking on. What you can do is learn to manage your activities better so that you use your time more effectively. Busy people everywhere may feel they are not using their time effectively. The more predictable, routine and consistent the work the easier it is to manage effectively, for jobs are done again and again with little disruption. If the work involves few or no other people it is also easier to manage because there will be fewer interruptions and less variation to your pattern of behaviour.

Unfortunately health care is not like this. Some of the procedures may be routine, some of the activities may be consistent and predictable, but the most significant variable relates to the fact that it is a *people business* and people are not predicable, routine and consistent. Health care is a dynamic business, involving many people at many different levels and in many different categories. Human behaviour is not easy to predict and not easy to plan for. People's health needs vary and their perception of their health needs also varies. Their satisfaction levels vary and so do their demands.

The challenge for the health professional is to develop skills to be able to work as effectively as possible within the constraints of the environment and the reality of the industry and to learn to organise their work so that they have the resources and time available to respond to the unpredictable. In practical terms, this means to learn to:

- be clinically competent and confident
- utilise resources effectively
- avoid time-wasting behaviours (double handling, back-tracking, multiple levels of communication)
- recognise limitations
- locate and use resources when they are needed
- plan the day's activities and keep to routine as much as possible
- work within reasonable expectations
- anticipate change and disruption
- evaluate and review and modify behaviours: not do things the same way because that is the way they have always been done
- search out effective and efficient practices
- learn rather than judge: seek answers rather than people to blame.

There are usually staff development needs in all of those areas in any organisation. They will be expressed within work practice reviews and in everyday observation. No level of staff is immune to these needs and no individual has the answers all the time.

Occupational stress

The issue of *burnout* has probably received more attention than any other single problem concerning health care workers. It is often treated as a symptom of occupational stress and gives rise to staff turnover and loss of people from health professions. Burnout can be perceived as a symptom of the profession. Any situation can be a challenge to one individual and a source of stress to another. For any individual this can change with different situations and at different times. The situation may not be the problem but is the individual's response to the situation that causes the concern and it is in the area of response where a great deal of staff development may be needed.

Stress has been described as the disease of this century and the cause of many of the physical and behavioural illness of today. Individuals, including health care workers, have been feeling the physical and psychological effects of a stressful situation since the beginning of time, not just in this century. The source of stress is within the outside world and it is the individual's ability to respond to and deal with a situation that results in a feeling of concern to a lesser or greater degree.

Health care professionals frequently describe their work as *stressful* and identify stress as an occupational hazard. Contact with other professionals as part of personal and professional development programs has led me to believe that the single most significant source of stress is the individual's response to the *expectations of their role*. Expectations of performance may be unrealistic. Expectations are placed upon or felt by the individual from:

- themselves as a professional
- the profession of which they are a member
- the community/client for which they provide a service

It is how the individual deals with those expectations that can decide how they feel about their job and the extent to which they feel stressed or burnt out.

Cooper and Marshall (1976) in Donovan and Jackson (1991) cluster potential sources of stress into six major categories. What becomes clear is that organisational factors and the quality of management can play a large part in what stress is generated and managed in health care.

Common sources of occupational stress

Factors intrinsic to the job	working conditions
	work load
	shift work
The role of the organisation	role ambiguity
	role conflict
	responsibility for people
	other role stresses
Relationships at work	relationships with superiors
	relationships with subordinates
	relationships with colleagues
Career development	career profession problems
	status incongruity
Organisational structure and climate	worker involvement in organisational processes
Extra organisational factors	work/home factors
	dual career factors
	(especially for women)

The staff development needs from these factors are obvious. Staff development initiatives can be at different levels (Green 1982):

- professional and educational interventions
- organisational interventions
- management interventions
- individual interventions.

In summary, staff development needs can arise from many areas of the work place and can be different for every individual employee. However, this section has identified common themes that can provide a useful framework for further needs assessment and for program planning.

Chapter summary

Needs assessment is an integral part of planning for staff development. It does not end with the collection and analysis of data but extends into the program planning phase, guiding the selection of solutions to staff development needs. An essential component of planning in staff development is a systematic, relatively objective way of assessing needs in order to make decisions about priorities for services or programs. The purpose of needs assessment is not to suggest solutions but to identify those areas where solutions are most required and to set criteria for their solution. This chapter has looked at the purpose of needs assessment in health care in terms of the creation of a three-way partnership between the service provider, the service receiver and the stakeholder in the organisation. Four common methods of conducting a needs assessment were outlined—interview, questionnaire, observation and workshop. As questionnaire is the most common, a detailed description of the development of a questionnaire was outlined. Finally, planning staff development based upon needs was outlined. Common areas or need were classified into three areas—the update of clinical experience, work load management and occupational stress.

REFERENCES

Beach E K 1984 Johari's window as a framework for needs assessment. Journal of Continuing Education in Nursing 13(3):28-32

Donovan F, Jackson A C 1991 Managing human service organisations. Prentice Hall, Sydney

Green D 1982 A framework for considering the burnout syndrome. In: Boss P, Smith N (eds) Professional burnout. Monograpy 2, Monash University, Melbourne

Horner B 1991 Needs assessment for staff development in the Silver Chain Nursing Association. University of Western Australia Press, Perth

Hunt J W 1986 Managing people at work: a manager's guide to behaviour in organisations. McGraw Hill Book Company, London

Kristjanson L J, Scanlan J M 1989 Assessment of continuing nursing education needs: a literature review. The Journal of Continuing Education in Nursing 20(3):118-123

Punch K, Horner B 1990 Stages in the development of a needs assessment questionnaire. Journal of Nursing Staff Development 7(4):176-180

Van Schoubroeck L 1986 The GHQ: a psychometric analysis. Department of Education, University of Western Australia

Witkin B R 1984 Assessing needs in education and social programs. Jossy Bass, San Francisco

3

Elements of learning and teaching

Key questions

- Do different people learn in different ways?
- On what principles of learning do you base your teaching?
- Do adult learners learn differently?
- What is your most effective teaching style?

Content summary

Introduction

Theories of learning
  Stimulus-response theory
  Cognitive learning theory
  Humanistic theory
  Systems theory

Accelerated learning theory

Principles of learning
  Perception
  Environment
  Problem solving
  Prior learning

Principles of learning specific to the adult learner

Principles of teaching
  Rapport
  Communication
  Learning needs
  Objectives
  Planning
  Evaluation

Teaching methods
  Informal teaching
  Structured teaching
  Supervision/preceptorship
  Competency-based teaching

References

Introduction

It is very difficult to talk about teaching or learning without reference to the inter-relationship between the two. One teaches because someone needs to learn and one learns because someone teaches.

However, it is a mistake to assume that an individual only learns when a teacher is present or that because you are a teacher someone will learn. I have heard individuals say, 'What a great teacher, he really kept me entertained. Mind you, I don't know if I learnt anything'. I have also heard individuals say, 'That was a great session. Everything went according to my plan and I really enjoyed myself.' This individual has had a *good teach*. In neither case can you be sure that learning has occurred, but certainly, some teaching went on. You could ask, whose needs are being met?

This chapter aims to provide information that if applied, will ensure that the needs of both the learner and the teacher are met. The information and examples will provide a foundation upon which your expertise as a teacher can be built because you will develop as a *learner-centred teacher*. In this way both learner and teacher can benefit.

Theories of learning

Learning is a very personal process. No two people necessarily learn the same way, nor does one individual learn the same way all the time. There are, however, some principles against which the process of learning can be examined.

Learning can be seen as a process by which changes are brought about in an individual's *response* to a given situation. An individual will respond in the way they have found most effective for learning. This response, although the individual may not realise it, is based upon a *way of learning* or learning theory. Studying theories of learning is a discipline in itself and many books have been written on the topic. You may find this topic very interesting and may choose to pursue it in far greater depth than will be discussed here. For the purpose of understanding your learners better, a brief explanation of some of the more useful theories of learning is presented here. With each theory, the implications for teachers will be identified.

Stimulus-response theory

Stimulus response theory is based on experimental findings that behaviour can be provoked through specific stimuli and reinforced by rewarding the desired behaviour. Put simply, if you reward positive behaviour it will be repeated. This simple method of learning is common in young children when behaviour is simply rewarded and/or punished. It does not encourage thoughtful interaction or participation in the learning process but rather encourages a response that can become automatic with practice. For example, mice can be taught to follow the maze by repeated positive reinforcement. In the same way pigeons have been taught to peck when a light comes on, for which they get fed. The application of this theory to teaching is mainly on arranging stimuli, providing cues and reinforcing the desired response. Many clinical skills taught to a student nurse in the early stages of a program, may involve the application of this theory of learning. Clinical situations where an immediate or automatic response is required may be taught this way so that the behaviour becomes *second nature*.

The learner may not question or challenge what is being taught but rather accept it as what is expected of them in terms of behaviour.

Teaching principles derived from the stimulus-response theory are as follows:

- The learning situation is best arranged so that the learner is active and able to respond quickly.
- Concepts are presented in simple context.
- Response comes with recognition of the stimuli as well as learned behaviour.
- Appropriate behaviour is reinforced.
- Repetition and practice of responses is encouraged.
- The teacher tends to function as a trainer not facilitator of learning.

Cognitive learning theory

Cognitive learning theory views learning as a perceptual and conceptual process which modifies the person's knowledge base and structure. It implies that the individual thinks about both what they are learning and how they are learning (cognition). It involves the acquisition of knowledge and understanding and development of mastery over new knowledge. Central to cognitive learning theory is the acquisition of facts. A process occurs where the learner connects new knowledge with old knowledge, sometimes replacing the old with the new, but sometimes building onto the old. The learner seeks to understand the information rather than just accepting it and needs to find meaning in what they are learning. The learner seeks to understand what is being taught and may have difficulty learning something they can not make sense of.

Teaching principles derived from cognitive learning theory are as follows:

- Central key facts are presented.
- Learning is designed to be systematic, starting with the simple and building to the complex, thus facilitating the development of knowledge.
- Learners are encouraged to challenge and ask questions.
- Learners are encouraged to set individual learning goals defined in terms of information content.
- Divergent and convergent thinking is facilitated to accommodate learners who expand to view the big picture as well as learners who seek to pull concepts together.
- The teacher facilitates learning and comprehension rather than just presenting.

Humanistic theory

Humanistic theory takes a global view of the learner, that is, it considers the learner within his/her environment, recognising that there may be psychological, sociological or cultural aspects that will influence the learning process. Learning is not viewed in isolation. It is seen as a process of discovering how the learner relates to people, things and ideas within his/her total life situation and how the information may influence any of these relationships. For example, the information I may present as a teacher may be absolutely crucial for you to know. But if the information I am presenting, or the behaviour I am seeking to bring about is in conflict with your cultural beliefs, it is unlikely that you will be able to internalise and adopt that behaviour, no matter how important you see it to be.

Humanistic learning theory is sometimes seen as only appropriate in behavioural subjects where there may be an expectation of psychological understanding and rapport. However, if you have ever tried to study statistics, when you have had experience in a school system where you believed (or your results indicated) you were *hopeless at maths*, or where it was seen that *girls could not do maths*, you will understand how cultural and social experience can influence your ability to learn. Within humanistic theory, it would be recognised that it was important that you work through some of those old patterns and messages before you could learn with an open mind.

Teaching principles derived from humanistic learning theory are as follows:

* The teacher's role is to facilitate learning not teach directly.
* Individuals learn only if they perceive the information to be relevant to their own existence and surroundings.
* Experience which involves a change to self is resisted.
* Learning occurs more freely when individuals are relaxed and not under threat.
* Learning never occurs in isolation.
* A relationship of trust and respect will enhance learning.
* Past experiences will always influence learning.

Systems theory

Systems theory has been developed from an understanding of biological systems and from the application of biological principles to social situations. A system is a set of dynamic interdependent parts and a change in one component is transferred throughout the system until a readjustment is made.

A system functions in terms of input, output and feedback. The input is the stimulus to the system, the output is the product which the system is designed to produce, while feedback is the communication within the system whereby one component is connected to another.

Applied to systems theory of learning, this means that new information presented to a learner will interact with all other relevant information the learner may currently have until the learner finds a way to *fit* the information into a pattern of knowledge. All the pieces or parts to the knowledge will interact with other pieces or parts and try to *fit* together. The parts of the system are the new knowledge (input), the required behaviour (output) and the relationship between the parts (feedback).

Examples of a social system include a ward, a school, a hospital, a family and a football team. Changes made by one member of the system is likely to affect other members of the system. We know this happens in families and sporting teams, where the behaviour of any one individual can influence all the other members. In terms of a body of knowledge it is a little harder to see the connection, but it can be recognised that knowledge is inter-related and new knowledge in one area can influence knowledge in another area.

Teaching principles derived from systems theory are as follows:

- Behaviour change as a result of teaching and learning is only one component of an individual's life and this new behaviour could be influenced by another component.
- Attitudes and knowledge relating to such things as home life, religion and politics are all interrelated and can affect each other so that knowledge in any one area may influence behaviour in another area.
- Education in a specific area may lead to a complex process of change and adjustment in many aspects of one's life, which may be harmful as well as beneficial.
- Learning in one area can influence existing knowledge in another, possible unrelated area.

Accelerated learning theory

Accelerated learning theory has three key principles (Rose 1985):

- Learning is influenced by the energy wave state of the brain.
- Learning involves the whole brain.
- Learning is influenced by multiple levels of intelligence.

Learning is influenced by the energy wave state of the brain

The energy that naturally runs through the brain is divided into four different brain wave states:
Delta state: deep, dreamless sleep, 0.5-3.5 cycles per second
Theta state: dream state, accessed for meditation, creativity and for direct healing, 3.5-7 cycles per second
Alpha: relaxed state, rate used for programming, 7-13 cycles per second
Beta: conscious, active, 13-28 cycles per second.

It is interesting to note that in the beta state we can think of up to nine things at a time and, it is the only state of stress within the brain. Between the conscious and unconscious mind there is a filter which is part of the reticular activating system of the brain. This filter is open in the alpha state and tightly closed in the beta state. It is the alpha and theta states where we can get access to the subconscious mind, that is, the memory, which is about 88% of the mind. Therefore, in learning the aim is to access and utilise the subconscious mind to program information. The key is that the mind must be relaxed; a calm brain learns best. The application of this is obvious. People under stress do not learn well and conversely, learning is most effective when the mind is relaxed. That is why music is such an effective learning medium to create a relaxed learning environment. Research has shown that the heartbeat adjusts to music. For the majority of people, the relaxed state is a heart beat of between 56-64 beats to the minute. Playing music such as Baroque slows our heartbeat down to a relaxed (alpha) state where we can have single focused concentration and so learn more effectively.

Learning involves the whole brain

All individuals have the potential to use their whole brain for learning, that is, all their senses and both hemispheres of their brain. In terms of senses, an individual can learn by smell, touch, taste, hearing and sight. True learning involves all senses all the time in varying degrees. All senses form images which can be triggered in learning and can assist us to recall what we have learnt previously. If all of the senses can be involved, the learning is maximised. This calls for creative teaching but also makes learning more fun, more interesting and more likely to be successful. Left hemisphere learners often describe their learning style to be more logical, orderly, objective, linear and literal. They prefer such things as a sequence of numbers, repetition, verbalisation and often judge what they hear. Stereotypical examples of left brain learners are mathematicians, accountants and engineers. Men are often perceived to be predominantly left brain learners. In fact, research indicates 49.3% of men are true left and 26.0% of men are true right and the rest are a mixture of both.

Right hemisphere learners describe their learning style as imaginative, metaphysical, creative, spatial and holistic. They prefer such things as colour, pictures, visualisation, rhythm and stories. Stereotypical examples of right brain learners are musicians, artists and writers. Women are often perceived to be predominantly right brain, however, research indicates 35.1% are true left and 37.7% are true right and the rest are a mixture of both.

A useful tool is to remember this can be referred to as **VAKPOINT** learning where the letters refer to:

V = *visual learning*: visual learners prefer to see things; prefer pictures, diagrams and graphs

A = *auditory learning*: auditory learners prefer to hear things; prefer talking and music

K = *kinaesthetic learning*: kinaesthetic learners prefer to touch and feel things; prefer to have contact with material

PO = *print oriented learning*: print orientated learners prefer the written word; prefer to read and use books

INT = *interactive learning*: interactive learners prefer to learn with others; prefer to work in active groups.

VAKPOINT

V	= visual	use slides, overheads, pictures
A	= auditory	use music, your voice, discussion
K	= kinaesthetic	use touch and contact with materials
PO	= print oriented	use words, writing, handouts
INT	= interactive	use group work, exercises, shared activities

Learning is influenced by multiple levels of intelligence

We use seven different levels of intelligence to influence learning (Gardner 1993). These seven intelligences are:

1 *Mathematical/logical intelligence*: logical problem solving, planning details, experimenting, riddles, analysis; the why and how of learning
2 *Verbal/linguistic intelligence*: stories, proverbs, poetry, speeches, comedy, reading, metaphors, jokes
3 *Kinaesthetic intelligence*: exercise, drama, role play, mime, sports, crafts, dance
4 *Musical intelligence* : rhythm, music, drumming, language, musical instruments, humming, writing jingles, singing
5 *Visual/spatial intelligence*: imagination, colour, shapes, design, drawing, spatial models, mind charts
6 *Inter personal intelligence*: talking, communication, teams, groups, discussion, role play, listening
7 *Intra personal intelligence*: quietly relaxing, meditation, internal exploration.

Traditional learning institutions (schools, universities) use mathematical/ logical intelligence and verbal/linguistic intelligence. A more advanced approach will attempt to access all seven types of intelligence through a variety of learning and teaching strategies, according to the needs of the learners. It is an enormous challenge for the teacher, but the rewards for both learner and teacher are unlimited.

The application of this theory recognises that learning is multifaceted and calls for teaching to also be multifaceted. Individuals may have a preferred learning style, usually from habit rather than effect. The challenge for any learner is to relax the brain and activate both hemispheres of the brain so that learning can be captured by as many different styles and intelligences as possible (Howard 1991). Individuals who can learn to see things differently, and who are prepared to develop their learning tend to view the world in a new way and find talents they never knew they had. Learning can get blocked in one style but, with the exposure and stimulation, a different approach can be found. Similarly, learning can depend on one of the senses or an individual can become socialised into using one of the senses and not realise the joy of looking at something in a different way.

It is important to remember that in any one group of learners you will have individuals who *prefer* (have become used to) a type of learning. You can rarely reach all of the learners *all* of the time, but you can reach all of the learners *some* of the time if you vary the learning style. It is not difficult to think of ways of presenting material in all of the forms, but it is easy to forget and to fall back on the old well known styles, particularly print oriented and didactic presentation.

Teaching principles derived from accelerated learning theory are as follows:

- Within any group there will be individuals with all preferred learning styles.
- Material should be presented in all styles at some time in any one session if you want to capture all individuals some of the time.
- Learners will grasp onto their preferred style but can still tune into other styles if the material and presentation is integrated.
- Teaching needs to be creative and innovative and is far more fun.
- Teachers will tune into their own style along with those of the learner.

In summary, it would be useful to consider these theories in terms of the way you *like* to do things, that is, your preferred learning style and be prepared to try different approaches to your work. Remember, your aim is to become a *learner-centred teacher,* so think of how you can turn your teaching sessions around to maximise the learning.

Principles of learning

The following principles may or may not be relevant in any given situation, or for any one individual. What is important is that the teacher recognises that learning may be influenced by many factors (Howie 1988).

Perception

Perception varies with anxiety, experience, motivation and interest. For example, I may *perceive* that a particular clinical skill is complex and feel frightened about making a mistake. Or I may *perceive* that my teacher is inflexible and demanding because someone else I work with tells me so. On the other hand, I may *perceive* that my performance is being judged by my ability to handle pressure rather than my knowledge and skill. I may respond to an opportunity to develop my ability to handle pressure as an evaluation of my poor performance.

The way we see a situation, that is, our perception of a situation, can be quite different from that of anyone else. Be cautious about presuming that the learner perceives either the material or the situation in the same way you do. Asking questions in the beginning is a good way to assess where the learner is at and to then take the opportunity to dispel misinformation or incorrect perceptions. Presenting clear objectives, asking for personal objectives, establishing clear outcomes and standards are all ways of establishing a common purpose, based on a clear perception.

Environment

The environment can be external and internal. Taking physical needs as an example of the external environment, they must be met before an individual can be receptive to learning. You may have experienced a situation when you felt tired, hungry, cold or hot, crowded or distracted by noise and unable to focus. The physical environment cannot always be changed but it can be managed well. For example, a very large room may be less than ideal, but you can arrange the seating so that it appears to be smaller. Hungry people can be fed a snack and a drink at the beginning of a session, to allow for mixing and discussion before the main part of the session begins.

Unfortunately, a great deal of work related learning (inservice or staff development) occurs when the physical environment is less than satisfactory.

For example, work may take place in a small room at the end of the ward, without teaching facilities like an overhead projector; or crammed into a ward office in the middle of a busy work area. Moving to a different environment, although it may take a little time, allows the learner to remove themselves from their work situation and to avoid, ignore or at least minimise distractions.

The internal environment is more difficult to manage but equally as important. How many of these situations can you relate to? A teaching session at the end of a shift when people are exhausted; after lunch when there is a mountain of work to finish for the day; immediately after lunch when everyone wants to take a nap. Learning takes energy and you do not soak up knowledge like a sponge. It takes energy to listen, process information, discuss, question and respond. Again, work related learning is often not *at the right time.*

It is useful to allow time to actually leave work outside. Distractions could be symbolically dropped into a box at the door. It is valuable to give learners permission to talk about unfinished business or work related business if they have things to get off the mind. Five minutes discussion could be allowed for pairs to talk about the day at the beginning of the session. It is important to give individuals permission to feel tired or distracted at first, but to then create new energy for your session. Five minutes relaxation could be encouraged followed by a shoulder massage to vigorous music.

Application

You plan to run a tutorial from 2.00–3.30 p.m. on a new technique that has been introduced. The learners have been at work all day and some have had to reorganise their work load to attend. If you start with talk and demonstration it is highly likely at least 25% will immediately fall asleep (or nod off and lose interest). You will have lost them for the whole session because they will never catch up even if they tune in later. If you start with a 15 minute non-threatening activity related to the topic, (brush up on their knowledge in a related area), or an unrelated activity to connect the group (games trainers play), there is a far greater chance of energising the learners and separating their work-related distractions from the learning at hand.

Active learning

Nobody likes to sit and listen for hours. True learning occurs in the first 15 minutes and falls to almost nil after 45 minutes of uninterrupted talk. The mind wanders, the seat becomes hard, the legs and neck become stiff and interest falls away. That is why it is so important to vary activities and involvement, to *mix it up,* so that interest can be recaptured before it is lost for good.

Internally, new knowledge must be assimilated and internalised if it is to remain with the learner. It is as if we need to do something with the information, to make it meaningful for us by applying it to a situation that will assist us to recall it later. Cognition, that is, understanding, is enhanced by activity and involvement in the learning process. We have all experienced situations when we thought we had mastered something - until we tried to do it. Memory is triggered by recall of the practical application of the learning to a relevant situation. Providing opportunities for the learner to try themselves out, with support and guidance, will increase the rate of retention and recall. It may be necessary to listen and watch for some of the time, but not all the time. Learning also occurs by watching others and assisting them to recall. Peer learning situations can be of great value and can enhance the learning of both parties.

Problem solving

The process of problem solving is a cognitive and behavioural activity that builds on knowledge. Concepts and mental pictures created during a problem solving activity will enhance learning and provide a template for a future situation. You may think it is more comfortable to work in predictable situations, to always know what is going to happen and to always have time to plan activities. In reality, however, when you are faced with a problem to solve and you solve it, you draw on information and apply it and your knowledge and understanding in that situation is consolidated.

Problems can be presented to the learner in many different ways. The more creative the situation, the greater the impact on the learner. Some examples are:

- a case study requiring the development of a care plan
- the identification of errors within information
- a series of situations that can only be resolved with successful answers
- a group activity requiring team work to solve a problem
- a hypothetical scenario requiring thinking on your feet
- an interactive computer-based case study which leads the learner through the solution.

Learners may appear to want you to present the material to them on a platter, but they will benefit far more if given a problem to solve which involves the application of their knowledge.

Prior learning

A truly disadvantaged learner is one who is made to feel he or she knows nothing, or that everything they knew is out of date or useless. No previous knowledge is completely useless. Everything we learn is based upon past experiences and any knowledge or skill can be the foundation upon which new learning can be built. If the learner is made to feel nothing they know is of value, or that it has all become obsolete, they may lose confidence in their ability to learn anything new.

Knowledge today changes faster than we can forget. Most information has a half-life of about five years, which is not very long at all. This does not mean it should be discarded but rather that it requires updating. It may need modification or parts may need discarding, or the learner may need assistance to get out of old patterns. It can however still be useful and relevant.

No one likes to feel devalued or unrecognised. A learner who is made to feel devalued and insecure with messages that their knowledge level is no longer relevant will close off from learning. Their energy goes into responding to their feelings and surviving the emotional dislocation they feel. Certainly it is difficult for some people to let go of past behaviours and patterns and at times this difficulty can restrict new learning. But the individual needs to be assisted to feel comfortable again with the new knowledge level. This may result in less confidence and some insecurity at first.

Principles of learning specific to the adult learner

Learning has no age barrier; neither does our ability to learn decrease with age. Certainly, our learning may be influenced by other factors and our learning skills may need refreshing, but the ability to learn does not decrease.

The adult learner tends to be experience-laden, now-oriented, goal-directed and individualistic. As most learners in work settings are adult learners, it is useful to recognise some principles of learning specific to the adult learner (Zemke & Zemke 1988).

- The adult learner does not always learn for the love of learning, therefore learning must be relevant and meaningful.
- Theory needs to be integrated into practice.
- Learning is most effective if it can be applied to the work setting.
- The adult learner tends to take errors personally and is more likely to let errors affect their self esteem.
- Frequent feedback is essential as adult learners need to know how they are doing.
- The adult learner often holds unrealistic expectations of themselves and needs help to set realistic goals.
- The adult learner prefers teachers who act as facilitators rather than instructors.

- The adult learner tends to be outcome-oriented and look for results of their work.
- Adult learners are very supportive of each other.
- The adult learner often views assessment as a measurement of them as individuals not of their work.
- Adult learners can be self-directed in their learning, but that does not mean they do not need support.

The teacher may need to modify their approach for adult learners if they are going to facilitate learning effectively. Here are some strategies that may be useful to remember.

Useful strategies for adult learners

- Take time to get to know the learner and to find out what is going on in their life and to appreciate that considerable juggling may have gone on to get to this session. The learner is likely to come to a session with a million other things on their mind. This is not necessarily a lack of interest, but may be just a reflection of what else they are currently involved in.
- Show application early and mix theory with practice. The adult learner will seek relevance to their work situation in what they are learning and will have difficulty learning something just because it is good to know. They will want to apply it immediately.
- Expect harsh judgement and criticism and be prepared to help the learner to put things into perspective. The adult learner judges themselves harshly easily and may get discouraged and disillusioned quickly if they feel things are difficult to grasp.
- Provide an opportunity for demonstration of knowledge or skill early and make a point to acknowledge performance and effort. The adult learner needs feedback early and frequently to use as benchmarks for their performance.
- Work to find common threads within a group and link learners together in activities where they can develop supportive relationships. The adult learner benefits by seeing that there are others like themselves.
- Always acknowledge previous knowledge and experience and find ways for this to be demonstrated as a foundation for new information

Principles of teaching

Principles of teaching are derived from principles of learning; that is, effective teaching is based either directly or indirectly on the way people learn. Therefore, the teacher is guided both generally and in specific situations by the characteristics of the learner and their preferred learning style. The skilful teacher can modify a session on the run to meet the needs of the group.

There are a number of principles that form a foundation for effective teaching.

Rapport

Rapport will establish the climate for learning. For example, if a learner feels respected and accepted he or she will ask questions and feel relaxed and open to learning. If a teacher aims to get to know the learner as an individual, to recognise their particular characteristics and traits, the teacher will be able to design their teaching around the characteristics of the learner. The ability to create a rapport with the learner can be affected by prejudice, stereotyping, past experiences, your own level of confidence and experience and the feedback you receive. If learners see that the teacher is also open to learning about them as individuals or by recognising their past experience and knowledge, then respect for the teacher will develop.

Communication

Teaching involves a communication process and the principles of effective communication apply in all teaching situations. In verbal communication the medium of exchange is language; therefore, the receiver must know what meaning the sender attaches to the words that are used. It is essential to define terms so that the meaning is clear. This refers to technical terms within the context of the information and to general terms. For example, two people can have a different meaning for the term *competent* or *mastery*. Or, the teacher's understanding of terms like *goals* or *criteria* may be different from that of the learner. So much time can be wasted when two people think they are communicating effectively but where, in fact, they have not established a common language. Think of the number of times you have said, *Oh, I thought you meant ...*

Nonverbal communication, often unconscious behaviour, can have a marked effect on communication. Although people are often aware of other people's nonverbal communication, they may have never examined their own. Nonverbal communication means such things as facial expression, gestures, tone of voice, eye movement and body position. A learner can be encouraged by a nonverbal expression even though nothing is said and their ability to learn can be affected. In teaching, communication is a major component of the role and most teachers become expert in the art of nonverbal communication to encourage and lead a learner on in conversation. This art of effective communication will make the difference between a teacher who delivers a message and one who ensures learning will occur.

Learning needs

The greatest mistake a teacher can make is to assume they know what the learner's needs are. Teaching what someone already knows or what you *think* they should know, is wasteful of time and energy and can close the learner to future learning. In preparing the material, the teacher may have have a good understanding of the required outcomes for a session, or be aware of new information that must be presented to teach a new skill or technique, and so meet their needs as a teacher. This in itself is not enough to ensure learning. The teacher must remain open to modifying the session to meet the needs of the learner if they find gaps in assumed knowledge or that the situation has changed for the learner. An assessment of the situation can be made quickly at the beginning of the session and an invitation can be given to learners to tell the teacher what they feel their learning needs are. Simple techniques include asking questions, listening, observing reactions to what is said and remaining tuned into the audience.

A teacher may feel they have had what could be called *a good teach* when they have been tuned into what they were doing, rather than to what is happening for the learner. There is nothing wrong with enjoying what you are doing and leaving a session feeling positive and satisfied with the outcome. It is good to recognise that you have done a good job. But the success of the session may have only met your needs as a teacher and not the needs of learners. The greatest success comes when both teacher and learner feel the session has been successful and enjoyable. (See Ch. 2 for a detailed discussion of needs assessment.)

Objectives

Clearly stated objectives are an essential component of all teaching. The intended outcome of the session determines the content, that is, you must know where you want to go so that you can work out how to get there. Objectives relate directly to what the learner needs to know. They also become the basis of evaluation because you evaluate the outcome against the objective. Teachers may also have objectives that relate to their teaching. For example:

- to utilise more pictures and graphs to explain concepts
- to provide an opportunity for all participants to become involved
- to use clear overheads.

The content of the session, however, is written in terms of the learner's objectives. For example:

- to explain in their own words the way to bring about change
- to identify all the components of an infusion pump
- to develop a teaching plan for a session on safe sex practices.

Without clearly defined objectives, the session runs the risk of losing focus and not achieving the required results. It is important that objectives be written in a clear and precise fashion ensuring that there is no doubt about what an objective means or implies. An objective is based on action; that is, the learner will be able to do something with the information presented to them. Therefore, an objective needs to make a statement that can be achieved, a measurable outcome. Examples of words that can be used in an objective are: write, recite, identify, differentiate, solve, construct, list, compare, contrast. In clinical terms, words that can be used in an objective include: to demonstrate, to perform, to illustrate, to select.

When writing objectives, the following template is useful. It can be part of the objective or it can be a silent prompt. Keep the words simple and restrict each objective to one outcome. When you write an objective, ask yourself the question, *how can this be measured?* For example, how can you measure that someone can understand something, or reflect upon something. Take a look at these objectives:

Objectives

At the end of this session, the learner will be able to:
- show by return demonstration the correct procedure for an abdominal dressing
- demonstrate between passive and active exercises
- describe the difference between health teaching and health promotion
- list the muscles of the pelvic floor
- identify six principles of effective teaching.

Planning

Any teaching session should begin with a plan. When teaching is still new to you, planning is more important than presentation. With experience, the planning can become less formal and can be seen as a guide rather than a formal structure. A teaching plan should include the following components:

- clear statement of purpose often represented by the title
- clearly defined realistic objectives
- introduction including an overview
- organised sequential content developed in chunks or bite size pieces
- summary and review
- method of evaluation or feedback for learners and for the teacher
- details of the strategies and methods to be used.

A plan can always be modified or refined during a session as the session evolves or as you get to know the learners better and changes should be anticipated and accounted for. Few teaching sessions go absolutely to plan but a session that has no plan can be a disaster for teacher and learner.

Evaluation

Evaluation is an essential part of learning and teaching. Both learner and teacher need detailed and constructive feedback and need to look beyond an intuitive sense or gut feeling that an outcome was achieved. Evaluation can be seen as a planned continuous process of obtaining feedback. Some common evaluation techniques are oral questioning, questionnaire surveys, checklists, rating scales, written tests, diaries, process recordings and audits.

Educationalists distinguish between *formative* and *summative* evaluation. *Formative evaluation* applies to a continuous process of feedback throughout the learning and teaching situation. This helps to determine the pace and extent of learning and allows the teacher to vary the process to meet learners' needs. Examples include a question and answer break within the session, inviting someone to explain their understanding of information to the group, a return demonstration and a check-list to take away as review for the next session. *Summative evaluation* applies to a process conducted at the end of a session to determine what has been learned. Common examples include written and oral examinations, practical examinations and assignments.

Comprehensive evaluation will encompass structure, process and outcome to analyse the total picture. *Structure* concerns itself with aspects of the environment including the availability of premises, expertise and equipment. Questions to guide structural evaluation might be:

- What topics were dealt with?
- Which staff were involved?
- Were the facilities and resources adequate?
- Was there enough time?
- Was the environment conducive to learning?

Process evaluation concerns itself with how resources were used, what types of techniques were employed and how appropriate were these resources and techniques in relation to the particular learners and the learning task at hand.

Questions to guide process evaluation include:

- Were the learner's perception of his or her needs elicited?
- Was the learner involved in the learning method?
- How did the learner participate?
- Was the teacher credible to the learners?
- Was the interaction active and was discussion allowed?

Outcome evaluation is involved with end results. A desired outcome may be defined as a change in behaviour, an increase in knowledge, a shift in attitude and/or behaviour. Outcome evaluation is directly related to the objectives set for the session and if they are clear and measurable, then outcome evaluation will be meaningful. It is unrealistic to evaluate an outcome that was not identified in the objectives. Questions to guide outcome evaluation include:

- What were the changes in knowledge and/or behaviour?
- Was there evidence of an increased ability to analyse, participate and adapt behaviour?
- Can they demonstrate understanding through the integration of all the relevant facts?
- Did the methodology achieve the desired results?
- Have the objectives been met?

Evaluation techniques gather information which, when interpreted, can show if and how learning has occurred. As mentioned, the techniques must be designed to measure the kind of learning specified in the objectives. The techniques must also be *valid* and *reliable*. *Validity* means the technique measures what was intended to be assessed. For example measuring the ability to demonstrate passive exercises with a written test is not a valid technique. *Reliability* refers to the consistency of a measurement tool, which should generate consistent responses provided there has been no interference or intervention in the meantime. For example, an examination that produces marked variations in results between homogeneous groups may be unreliable. A practical examination when conditions are inappropriate may produce an unreliable measure of ability.

Evaluation provides feedback: feedback for the learner which will motivate and guide learning; feedback for the teacher which will indicate strengths and areas needing improvement and can provide job satisfaction; feedback for the employer/manager which can help to identify effective outcomes and needs for future processes.

Teaching methods

Over time, you will probably develop a teaching style that best suits you. Some styles will feel confortable and others will not. Regardless of your preferred style, which is often just what you have got used to, it is useful to review and trial other styles. Remember that the aim is to use a style that is most effective for the group, not just what feels comfortable to you.

Teaching methods can be organised into broad categories. The method of teaching you choose for a particular group depends on several factors, such as the nature of the subject matter, the nature of the learner, the facilities and/or environment, the size of the group, or the desired outcome.

Informal teaching

Informal teaching tends to be somewhat unstructured or casual and can take place almost anywhere. It might be on the spot in response to a question, initiated by the learner without any planning by the teacher, or it may take place without either party realising learning is going on. This does not mean it is unimportant or unstructured and all the principles of teaching still apply. Activities may include talking and listening, asking and answering questions, or setting an example. Informal teaching goes on all the time at work, such as between two work mates where one becomes the teacher for the other. There may be little time for planning but the outcome can still be very successful. Adult learners often feel very comfortable with an informal style because it feels more collegial and less threatening.

Structured teaching

Structured teaching is planned well in advance according to a definite teaching guide or outline and scheduled for a specific time and place. All the techniques mentioned in informal teaching can be used, but they are planned rather than accidental. The most common methods of structured teaching are discussion, debate, lecture, demonstration, workshop and tutorial. Preparing for a structured teaching session should involve the following steps:

- Clearly identify the desired outcome.
- Write clear objectives.
- Develop the content into sections or 'chunks' in line with the objectives.
- Establish a time frame which allows time planned for each section.
- Identify the tools or aids you intend using such as overhead projector, white board, flip charts, charts and diagrams, music, slides, audio visual equipment and computers.
- Select activities to be included such as group discussion, questions, peer reporting, demonstration, observation.
- Develop a powerful beginning to get their attention and a 'punchy' ending to send them away with a memory.
- Develop an evaluation strategy and/or testing method.

Supervision/preceptorship

Supervision is a process where an expert or more experienced practitioner guides and directs the performance of a less skilled practitioner in order to help and improve their performance. Supervision implies 'watching over' to some people, but this is not the intent. Certainly there is an element of responsibility for the learning that takes place and often the learner needs to be watched. However, the relationship between the two parties is more collegial and often both parties learn from each other.

In nursing for example, supervision is now better known as *preceptorship* or *peer teaching*, providing the teacher/guide is at a more advanced level of expertise. It has become a common practice for newly graduated nurses to work with a preceptor for a period of time while they develop confidence and consolidate knowledge and skills. The preceptor becomes a mentor, sounding board, adviser, and sometimes confidant, as well as a teacher. It is a demanding role and takes time and energy to do well. It takes the preceptor away from their primary role at times and planning for this type of learning should incorporate a lesser work load for the preceptor. The preceptor becomes a catalyst for learning and the role is one of a true facilitator.

Supervision/preceptorship is made more effective by a cooperative relationship, good knowledge of the work involved, skilful communication and constructive evaluation. It requires good interpersonal skills as well as an advanced level of knowledge and expertise. Frequent feedback is a key component of this type of learning and there is a need for thoughtful, constructive praise and sometimes criticism. Adult learners respond particularly well to a supervisor/preceptor because they feel they can develop a relationship and interact on a personal level. The learner feels the learning and teaching is individual.

Competency-based teaching

Competency-based learning and teaching is the national agenda for training in Australia in the 1990s. Training bodies and professional groups have grasped onto the concept seeing it to be *the* way to quantify and evaluate performance. This is true to a certain extent. However, the application of competency-based learning and teaching is complex and involves a fundamentally different way of thinking for some people. It requires careful analysis of what one does and the identification of what one does that is different from any one else. It calls for critical assessment which is often perceived to be quite threatening. Competency-based learning and teaching is very useful, but it is only one method. It has unfortunately become rather like a crusade for many people and is supported with rigid commitment.

A *competence* is an attribute of a person which results in effective and/or superior performance. Competence comprises specification of knowledge and skill and the application of that knowledge and skill to an established standard of performance required for a position. *Descriptors* are statements which set down the properties that characterise something of the expected standard of performance. A cue (exemplar) is a selected concrete example of an activity that demonstrates the competence. The concept of competency includes all aspects of performance including:

- performance at an acceptable level of skill
- organisation of tasks
- responding and reacting appropriately when things go wrong
- fulfilling a role in the scheme of things
- the transference of skills and knowledge to new situations.

National competencies have been developed for nursing. Each competency is described in terms of the domain of performance, the required competency and a cue, or example, of how that competency can be demonstrated.

Competencies for a registered nurse

Domain	*Professional and ethical practice*
Competency	*Demonstrates a satisfactory knowledge base for safe practice*
Verbal description	*Demonstrates an accurate and comprehensive knowledge*
Cue	*Identifies theoretical concepts and principles underlying clinical practice*

Australian Nursing Council Inc (ANCI) 1993

Clearly, some competencies for some skills are easier to write than others and competencies to demonstrate behavioural areas of performance are quite difficult. Competency-based learning and teaching does provide an opportunity for clear recognition of prior learning, often presented in training circles as steps in a career pathway which allows for sequential movement through levels. Competencies have become the components of multi-skilled performance and may be referred to as the requirements for a position.

The development of competencies allows for the formulation of standards, being the outcome of those competencies. For example, in nursing in Australia, *standards for nursing practice* have been developed which are recognised as the minimum standards required by the practitioner. These standards are based upon the *demonstration of competence* for practice, relevant to the level of nursing. They are written as *'the role and competencies of the registered (or enrolled) nurse'* and are circulated as the expected standards of practice for the beginning practitioner. Clearly, they facilitate an understanding of a common level of practice and make it quite clear to the learner what is expected of them and what they need to achieve. The process of confirming that a person has achieved competency is based on assessment. An assessment is made by observing examples of activities that illustrate competence.

The implications for the teacher in competency-based learning are:

- to develop clear competencies that are to be achieved
- to develop expected standards that will demonstrate performance (learning)
- to develop assessment strategies so that performance (learning) can be measured against a competency.

Teaching strategies

The choice of teaching strategy depends on the purpose or required outcome of the session. A significant part of teaching is entertainment and performance; that is, getting and maintaining interest, and keeping the audience with you. Any strategy that will capture interest and make a lasting impression can be used. Be creative, adventurous, different. Here are some examples of strategies that work:

- Play an active piece of music before the session starts and into the first few minutes to create a high energy level.
- Play a quiet piece of music when you have people discussing and sharing ideas to block out any uncomfortable silence and avoid overhearing among participants.
- Use humour and laughter to lighten up the situation, especially if you can use a personal example that will make you seem normal.
- Vary materials and teaching tools. For example, use some overhead slides, some handouts, read some material.
- Move people around to avoid sitting in the same position all the time.
- Encourage interaction and questioning.

Teaching strategies

To transfer knowledge
group discussion
group or individual exercises
lectures
forums
panel discussions
films, videos

To develop skills
demonstration of skills
role playing
peer teaching
programmed instructions

To practise problem solving
case studies
brain-storming
discussion groups
interactive activities
simulation
field trips

To change attitudes
debates
displays
pair interaction
free expression

Remember, for effective teaching:
The more you put out the more you get back

Chapter summary

This chapter aimed to present information about learning and teaching to provide a foundation upon which the expertise of a teacher can be built. The key has been to present a learner-centred teaching approach where the focus of teaching is upon the facilitation of learning. A number of theories, traditional and innovative, have been presented to demonstrate that individuals learn in many ways. Each learning theory may have its place, but the importance of identifying different learning styles has been emphasised. Various principles of teaching have also been presented with an emphasis on variety and stressing the importance of expanding expertise and experience. Finally, teaching methods and strategies were presented to provide examples of how teaching can occur.

REFERENCES

ANCI 1993 National competencies for the registered and enrolled nurse in recommended domains. Australian Nursing Council Press, Australia
Commonwealth of Australia 1993 Competency standards assessors. Design and Electronic Publishing by PSI Consultants, Canberra
Gardner H 1993 Frames of mind. Paladin, New York
Howard C 1991 All about intelligence. New South Wales Press, Sydney
Howie J 1988 The effective clinical teacher: a role model. The Australian Journal of Advanced Nursing, 5:2 18-23
Rose C 1985 Accelerated learning. Accelerated Learning Systems, England
Zemke R, Zemke S 1988 30 things we know about adult learning. Training July, 57-61

The staff development process

Key questions

- How can a staff development process be applied in the work place?
- What is the value of a staff development process for the employer?
- What is the value of a staff development process for the employee?
- How does staff development relate to performance management?
- What are common outcomes of the staff development process?

Content summary

Introduction

Staff development is an integral part of employment and equally as important to the employer as it is to employee. However, both employer and employee must perceive benefits from the investment of resources into a staff development process if the value is to be recognised. The organisation needs to see the relationship between staff development and performance of both individual employees and of the organisation as a whole. The management of performance through staff development then becomes the strategy to achieve the goals of the organisation. The integration of staff development within the total management of human resources, that is, the people and the importance of staff development in overall performance of the organisation, will become evident.

For a person new to a staff development role the magnitude of the task can be over powering at first especially if responsibilities extend to an entire department or the whole organisation. The role becomes more realistic and the outcomes more achievable when staff development is considered as a process and divided into manageable stages. To assist in the development of the role, key points in the implementation of each stage are presented using examples from actual experience.

The staff development process

Staff development has been defined in this book in this way:

> *A planned organised process of learning within an employment setting, designed to update or increase knowledge and/or skills or for personal growth and development, to improve performance or to meet advances or changes in direction or focus of a position or of an organisation.*

Within this definition staff development is described as a process, a series of activities that form part of a carefully designed and implemented process. This process was discussed in detail in Chapter 1 and the stages of the process are listed and summarised briefly again here.

Stages of the process reviewed

Stage 1: Recruitment

Recruitment aims to increase the likelihood of meeting the needs of the organisation with the selection of the best person for a position. It includes:

- development of job descriptions, roles and responsibilities for positions

- clarification of qualifications and experience for positions
- implementing marketing and advertising strategies
- identification of appropriate candidates from within the organisation and from outside.

Stage 2: Selection

Selection aims to choose the best applicant for a position using all the tools and strategies that are available. It includes:

- determining selection strategies such as resume, interview, references and assessment
- collation and review of information from candidates
- establishment of a selection panel
- development of guidelines for evaluating applicants
- consideration and review of information that is submitted with applications
- development of criteria and strategies for interviewing candidates
- establishment of strategies for determining a decision and for providing feedback to applicants.

Stage 3: Appointment

The formal appointment aims to establish a connection between the employer and employee within a contractual arrangement. It includes:

- offer of position to the successful applicant
- negotiation if necessary and if appropriate until agreement is reached
- agreement of a contract of employment
- establishment of an employment relationship between employer (the organisation) and the employee (the individual).

Stage 4: Orientation (ideally a minimum of one month)

Orientation occurs over a period of time and within a supportive environment and aims to introduce the employee to the requirements and expectations of the organisation and of his/her performance. It includes:

- orientation to the organisational structure, function, personnel, services and clients
- introduction to the position, place of employment and to colleagues
- establishment of supports and resources
- identification of immediate learning needs and setting of goals to meet those needs
- discussion of performance criteria and evaluation processes
- planned formal and informal education sessions.

Stage 5: Consolidation (ideally over a period of three months)

Consolidation aims to provide opportunities for the employee to increase confidence and competence in a position within an environment where immediate support resources become less formal. It includes:

- comprehensive understanding of the organisation and the position with greater emphasis on other parts of the organisation and outside influences
- continual review of performance
- review and reassessment of learning needs and established goals
- formal performance review.

Stage 6: Continuing education

The aim of continuing education is to provide opportunities for ongoing learning so that the needs of the employer and employee continue to be met. It includes:

- establishment of a planned process of ongoing education and development that addresses skills, knowledge and personal development
- ongoing review of learning and performance needs
- continual review of organisational and individual needs.

Stage 7: Promotion

Promotion aims to provide the employee with an opportunity for advancement and/or further development in response to the recognition of knowledge and ability. It includes:

- appointment to a new position
- period of orientation to, and consolidation for, the new position
- establishment of supports and resources
- identification of learning needs and setting of goals to meet those needs
- presentation of performance criteria and evaluation processes.

Stage 8: Exit

The aim at exit is to cease a contractual agreement of employment in the most satisfactory way for both employer and employee. It includes:

- submission of resignation or presentation of termination notice
- establishment of a mechanism for an interview, discussion or feedback session
- acknowledgment of the contribution made by employee.

Each stage has unique activities but the connection between stages is easy to see. Insufficient planning in one stage, or an unsuccessful outcome in another stage, can impact on some or all of the other stages. For example, the superficial analysis of the requirements for a position which results in a poorly defined job description, may result in the appointment of an individual whose performance does not meet the expectations of the organisation. If the individual is to stay in the position to which they have been appointed, the employer (the organisation) may find they have to provide considerable support and resources for the individual to consolidate his or her position and to invest further resources in continuing education. These extra demands may impact on other staff development activities. The results of a poor analysis of a position will be felt by the organisation and the individual for some time.

Value for the employer

To the employer, a staff development process will have benefit for the organisation and therefore benefit for the employees and clients. A staff development process can provide the employer with mechanisms for:

- establishing the culture of the organisation
- determining common standards for performance
- developing indicators to demonstrate performance
- realising opportunities for advancement and development
- establishing standards of care
- establishing standards for occupational health and safety
- building a climate for industrial relations
- identifying inefficiencies in performance
- managing change
- decreasing staff turnover and associated costs
- accommodating labour flexibility
- increasing job satisfaction
- identifying staff and client needs
- improving performance.

Implementing a staff development process enhances the likelihood of effective management of the human resources (the people) within an organisation.

Value for the employee

To the employee, a staff development process is evidence that the employer views his or her performance needs as relevant and important. A staff development process provides the employee with mechanisms for:

- understanding the culture of the organisation
- establishing common standards for performance
- measuring performance against established criteria
- identifying learning needs

- personal growth and development
- responding to change within the organisation
- realising job satisfaction
- career planning and development
- recognition
- participation in organisational goals and directions.

Application within a work place scenario

It may be difficult to visualise how the stages of the staff development process are linked together within a staff development program, or how responsibilities in each stage can be addressed at the same time as part of a staff development program. The following scenario and examples are presented to provide explanation.

Imagine you hold a nursing management position in a medium size day surgery clinic. Your management position includes responsibility for the nursing service and includes *staff development* for all fifteen nursing staff. You report to a General Services Manager (GSM) within the organisation but you have autonomy and the freedom to run your department as you see best. The staff are all registered nurses some of whom work full time but most work part time. The service is on site day surgery with some home visiting follow up service. The client group varies in age and their degree of need, dependent upon such factors as their age, home situation, nature of the surgery and general health.

You have been involved in the development of the clinic's goals and objectives and attend a monthly meeting with the General Service Manager, other departmental managers and other health professionals, to monitor the operation of the clinic. You in turn monitor your department in terms of:

- the nature of the surgery that is conducted
- the characteristics of the client population
- changes to procedures, technology and/or equipment
- the knowledge and skills of the nursing staff
- the working relationships between staff within your department and with other staff
- the morale of staff and the overall climate of the department.

You are alert for signs of negative stress among staff which may present in behaviour, attitudes or nursing practice. Your department's performance is measured by such things as the number of cases completed in a prescribed time period; satisfaction in the nursing care as indicated by clients, doctors and others; results from client satisfaction surveys; and functioning within budget. Your work seems to be increasing and even though you feel you are functioning well and you certainly enjoy your work, you have been feeling concerned that you are losing touch with your staff's needs as the management demands of your position take priority. You know that when it comes to managing your work, time spent in staff development activities slips to the bottom of the list.

It occurs to you that it may be useful to create a new position within the team, a team co-ordinator or team leader position. This position would take some of the staff development needs of your role from you and you in turn would be better able to manage your position more effectively. You decide to propose your idea to the General Services Manager who examines with you the financial and resource implications. It is agreed that the increase in salary costs that would result could be accommodated by a reorganisation of staff hours. The proposal is presented at the next general management meeting, including your rationale and the benefits to your department and to the clinic in general. You receive support in principle and explain that you would like to present the idea to the staff in the department at their next meeting.

At this meeting, you again obtain general support. You note one female nurse of many years experience, who seems to be strongly against the idea and you invite staff to talk to you individually about their concerns or ideas. Some staff do come and talk to you, including the one who seemed to have some concerns. In most cases you feel you were able to talk through any concerns and you gained a number of useful ideas. However, you do not feel sure that the staff member who was strongly against the idea has really changed her mind. The proposal is formed over the next days and you subsequently gain full support from management for the establishment of the position of *Team Co-ordinator, Nursing Services*. Nursing staff within the department indicate their further support during subsequent staff meetings.

Recruitment

You develop a job statement which includes a description of the role and the responsibilities of the position. You identify the qualifications and experience required for the position including such areas as clinical experience in day surgery, leadership ability, interpersonal skills, specific knowledge and experience in staff development. You review the current nursing staff to identify any possible candidates you would encourage to consider making application. It is agreed you will try to fill the position internally, but you still advertise the position externally, in the newspaper and in a day surgery newsletter. A copy of the advertisement is placed on the staff notice board and a copy is given to each staff member with their pay notices to make sure all part time staff see it. You receive three internal applications and two external applications. It seems to be general knowledge among staff as to who has applied from within the department.

Selection

Following discussion with management, the panel is selected to include yourself, the GSM and a nurse holding a position similar to yours in another day surgery clinic, with whom you have previously interviewed and whose contribution you value. You agree to review all applications in accordance with criteria you have determined and develop an interview schedule and strategy. You short list four of the five applicants (excluding one internal applicant who does not meet the criteria for interview) and interview them over one day. Staff in the department are aware of the interviews and you mentally note a sort of nervous energy within the clinic on the day. You note that the nurse who appeared particularly negative at the meetings had phoned in sick on the day.

Appointment

The panel makes a unanimous decision and you offer the position to one of the internal candidates, who accepts. This nurse has been working full time at this clinic for about two years and is considered one of the most experienced nurses in the department. The panel agrees that you will contact all the applicants and offer them a post interview meeting. The staff at the clinic are notified of the decision. The other internal applicant is disappointed but accepts the decision. You make a note to utilise her expertise more in the future. There are obvious advantages to making an internal appointment, but there are also disadvantages.

Internal appointment

Advantages	Disadvantages
Familiarity with the clinic	Lost opportunity for new ideas
Known by staff	Resentment of existing staff
Minimal associated costs	Role confusion can occur

In this scenario, this appointment is a promotion. A promotion to a new position does not alleviate the need for a period of orientation and consolidation. In fact it can be more important as the individual may need time to detach from the old role.

Orientation

You establish a one month orientation program with the Team Co-ordinator. It includes:

- introduction and development of the role
- reporting and communication lines and strategies
- changes from the old role
- identification of learning needs
- your expectations of the role

- her expectations of the role
- introduction of the new role to other staff
- working relationships with other staff.

You agree to convene a special staff meeting to give all staff the opportunity to hear the plans and to offer ideas and comments. At this meeting, most staff appear supportive and enthusiastic, although some cannot picture the new role at this time. The staff member whose attitude you had noted before as being particularly negative contributes little except to offer reasons why most things won't work. For example:

I don't know why this position was created—we don't need leading by anyone.
The best part about my job is being independent—I don't want anyone telling me what to do; and *I have been here the longest and I know what works well—everything is fine as it is.*

You and the Team Co-ordinator note the comments and the attitude and agree that the staff member needs an opportunity to talk about her concerns privately with you. You arrange an appointment at which you hope to identify the basis of the concerns, to assure her current position in the team, minimise any effect from her negative attitude on other staff and to elicit support by identifying her career goals and plans.

Not a great deal is achieved at the interview except to establish some base lines for performance in the future and to increase the understanding of the team co-ordinator position. It is obvious that this appointment cannot be considered in isolation, but rather has the potential to affect the entire team.

Consolidation

Over the next three months, the new position takes shape well and the Team Co-ordinator develops confidence with time and experience. The clinic staff in general and the clients adjust to the changes and you all begin to see benefits from the position. You are able to make some changes to your work practices and you feel you are managing your role more effectively. The needs of the team co-ordinator change over the three months, as do yours, as you learn to delegate and let go some of the areas and the staff development aspect of the new role develops. The staff member you interviewed continues to be challenged by the new situation and at times tries to undermine the position of the team co-ordinator. You still feel concerned and so decide to convene a meeting with the team co-ordinator and the GSM to discuss the situation. It is agreed that it is time for you to meet with the staff member again and this time to be more direct in stating what you are observing and your concerns.

Following a fairly intense interview in which there is some anger and frustration expressed by the staff member, you identify that she feels threatened by the team co-ordinator position, believes she should have been appointed and is preoccupied with personal problems. You reassure the staff member that she is a valuable member of your team but that you need to make your concerns quite clear. You offer the following opportunities. First, access to a staff counselling resource and second, attendance at a three day clinic on new techniques in day surgery to be held in the next month, if the nurse is prepared to work with you on her attitude and concerns. The counselling is received cautiously but the offer of the three day course is received with enthusiasm. You agree to meet in two weeks to assess the situation. You advise her that you will need to inform the team co-ordinator of the outcomes of the interview and the nurse accepts this.

You feel the situation may have been defused and that you may have redirected the nurse's energy into some more positive directions. There is no change over night but the nurse does appear less negative and at the next meeting, advises you that she has commenced counselling and would really like to attend the three day clinic. This is then arranged by the team co-ordinator.

Continuing education

The Team Co-ordinator conducts a staff needs assessment from which a program of staff development for the next six months is developed. The program consists of a variety of activities within a very flexible framework to allow all staff to organise the best way they can utilise the resources. The program includes the use of internal staff and some sessions accessing outside resources. The content has knowledge components, clinical skill components and personal de–velopment components. A program is also developed for the Team Co-ordinator and for yourself with the same flexible approach. The staff member who attended the three day course brings back to the centre new techniques and practices and begins enthusiastically to teach staff what was learnt. The nurse's expertise is acknowledged by other staff and, over time, this nurse develops the role of a clinical specialist in the team.

In summary

The process does not stop here. Over time, client needs or the demands of the service may give rise to further change in roles and/or positions. Another *promotion* may occur or a staff member may resign. With an *exit* interview you may identify other areas where change is needed. Constant monitoring of your role and performance and of the role and performance of the nursing staff in general will reveal which staff development program needs modification or alteration. Any staff development program should remain dynamic and flexible. What this scenario demonstrates is the relationship of the stages within the process and how a development in any one stage can influence another stage. The link throughout the process is performance management.

Performance management

The staff development process discussed here refers to an ongoing dialogue between employer and employee which comes with the establishment of an employment contract. The employer (the individuals' immediate manager) monitors the performance of employees and assists them to manage their performance through the identification of needs and implementation of strategies to address those needs.

Needs may be identified in terms of:

- the organisation/agency: they need staff with specific expertise in a particular area to provide the services offered by this agency
- the client population: it has become more multicultural and staff need to increase their awareness and understanding of the health needs of a different cultural groups
- the services: they have been modified in response to funding cuts and the staff need to develop expertise in some new areas
- the employees: changes in technology necessitate the development of new expertise, or the changes that are to be implemented will cause significant destabilisation of staff so you need to develop individuals as change managers to assist staff to adjust.

In all examples some common patterns emerge:

- an assessment of current performance was made
- findings were examined and interpreted
- a preferred behaviour or level of performance was identified
- a means of achieving the desired outcome or behaviour was determined.

By these means performance was managed.

The essentials of establishing a performance management system include setting clear objectives, obtaining commitment from all staff, overcoming resistance to change, involving participants in the development and design phases, conducting pilot tests, building in early successes and continual review and redesign. But the system begins with the premise that performance management is not an additional function or responsibility designed by the 'boss' but a systematic and effective system that is part of the total development of staff.

There are two occasions within employment when most needs are identified. They are within staff development activities such as a workshop and at the time of performance appraisal.

Performance appraisal

Performance appraisal is a formal system of measuring, evaluating and influencing the employee's performance; that is, skills, attitudes and behaviours (Guinn 1990). Its purpose is to discover at what level the employee is performing at a given time and to identify if the employee can perform more effectively or differently in a given period of time. It aims to be of benefit to the employee in terms of job satisfaction and to the employer in terms of outcomes.

Time and time again managers and their staff identify overwhelming dissatisfaction with an organisation's performance appraisal systems. Typical complaints charge that the systems are a waste of time at best, or destructive to staff relationships at worst. It may be the way the system is implemented or it may be the form that is used that causes the dissatisfaction. The fact remains, few organisations manage their performance appraisal system well and few staff view performance appraisal positively.

There are a number of potential positive outcomes of performance appraisal:

- performance measurement: the establishment of the relative value of an individual's contribution to an organisation based on measurement against established standards
- performance improvement: the encouragement of success and achievement and development in areas of need
- remuneration and benefits: determination of appropriate pay and bonus incentives based on merit results
- identification of potential: awareness of abilities
- feedback: outlining what is expected against actual performance
- communication: a format for constructive dialogue
- personal planning: the identification of goals based on realised need
- human resource planning: evaluation of supply and demand.

Performance appraisal is usually conducted annually or bi-annually. However, it is more effective if individuals receive ongoing feedback. If performance is being monitored and managed through out the year with ongoing feedback, the comments at an annual performance appraisal will be expected and accepted, rather than be the first time the individual has heard the comments. Performance appraisal requires the exercise of judgement and authority. In spite of the rhetoric about the scientific nature of a performance appraisal process, most decisions are based on a subjective judgement made by someone in a position of authority. To deny this subjectivity and judgement is at best unhelpful, and at worst destructive.

Conflict with performance appraisal is usually based upon problems of balance between one or all of the following:

- needs of the individual and the needs of the organisation
- quantitative and qualitative methodology
- objective and subjective judgements
- differences in the perception of standards
- differences in the perception of who should appraise
- differences in perception of the outcomes: what happens after an appraisal.

Organisations spend considerable time developing good performance appraisal forms, thinking that if they get a comprehensive form the results will be better. In fact, the form is possibly the least important aspect of performance appraisal. Some examples of forms can be found in the Appendix. The process of appraisal and the perceived benefits are far more significant than the form. Certainly the language and user friendliness of the form is important, but the form itself merely provides a guide for the interaction.

There are a number of methods of performance appraisal all of which aim to achieve a common outcome, such as measuring performance, identifying potential, giving and receiving feedback, planning the use of resources and facilitating communication.

Methods of performance appraisal

Essay technique	Appraiser writes a description of the individual's strengths and areas of need.
Advantage	in depth analysis
Disadvantage	time consuming; difficult to make comparisons
Graphic rating scale	Appraiser assigns a numerical value to each dimension indicating a rating range from superior to unsatisfactory performance.
Advantage	readily acceptable; more consistent.
Disadvantage	does not yield depth; validity can be challenged
Checklist	Appraiser records simple yes/no judgements on each dimension of performanc.
Advantage	expectations are clearly identified
Disadvantage	no degree or frequency of behaviour
Critical incident techniques	Incidents that are important are recorded and reviewed with the individual.
Advantage	the appraiser focuses on performance
Disadvantage	time consuming and difficult if incidents are not recorded accurately
Work standards techniques	Qualitative and quantitative work standards are set for a position.
Advantage	performance is measured, encourages employee participation.
Disadvantage	individual and organisation standards may not be the same
Assessment centres	Individuals are grouped together and assessed in a variety of ways; judgements are pooled and individuals are ranked and an order by merit ranking is assigned.
Advantage	particularly useful when individual's are not known; comprehensive
Disadvantage	costly and time consuming
Behavioural approaches	Scales are developed where each scale measures some job related behaviour.
Advantage	all aspects of performance are appraised
Disadvantage	problems with reliability; difficulty separating the person from the behaviour

To ensure success, regardless of the methodology used, it is important to answer first the following questions:

- What do I want to evaluate?
- What standards will I evaluate against?
- How do I want to evaluate: ratings, checklist, scores?
- What restrictions do I need to be aware of such as time, cost, staff numbers?
- What do I want the outcome of the appraisal to be: evaluation, selection, promotion, development or education?

Many organisations develop complex forms believing the more complex the form and the longer the time it takes to complete the assessment, the better the result. The opposite is usually true. Keep the form simple and easy to complete and spend most of the time discussing the results and their implications. The development of a form can be broken down into several steps.

Development of an appraisal form

Step 1   Identify key outcome areas
            List key areas outlined in the job statement
Step 2   List the behaviour(s) required to achieve the key outcome
            Identify more specific components of the position
Step 3   Develop criteria that will demonstrate achievement
            Identify actual behaviour that will demonstrate achievement
Step 4   Identify standards—statements of competence
            Identify top performance through to unsatisfactory performance and apply ratings (1 to 5)
Step 5   Develop indicators to demonstrate standards
            List actual behaviour for each criteria

Make sure there is plenty of opportunity for both the individual being appraised and the assessor (appraiser) to make comments, both in writing on the form and during discussion. Usually far more useful and meaningful information will come from comments, examples and discussion.

Performance indicators

Judgements of performance are usually based on the presence or absence of *indicators of performance*. A performance indicator can be described as a measure of achievement to assess performance in terms of effectiveness, efficiency and appropriateness (Mayo 1992). An indicator of performance assists an individual or an organisation to perform their work in the best way. Performed indicators are not a measure of activity (that is, how often something is done) but rather a measure of how well something is done. The three components are described as:

- effectiveness: measures the degree to which the objective is being achieved
- efficiency: measures the inputs and resources required to achieve a given objective or outcome
- appropriateness: measures if this is the best way to achieve the desired objectives or whether it could be done a better way.

Performance indicators are tools. They are not an end in themselves and should be viewed within the context of the situation in which they are being applied. Some useful rules for the use of performance indicators are as follows:

- Measure achievement not activity: how well have the objectives been met rather than how busy the individual is.
- Relate indicators to objectives: outcomes relate to objectives.
- Only apply indicators to activities within the individual's control. You cannot hold someone accountable for something not in their control.
- Express indicators numerically (1-5) against a previous score (benchmark) that was the level of performance indicated last time.
- Make indicators meaningful and useful: incorporate them into everyday performance.
- Recognise the significance of soft indicators: they are not absolute objective measures but only indicators.

Finally, it is useful to remember that individuals like to receive feedback, even if it is difficult to accept at the time. Employees can only measure their performance against those standards set by the organisation, the employer, and those set by their own values and standards. Individuals seek to perform well for their own intrinsic rewards as well as those of the organisation.

Examples of indicators

In the scenario of the day surgery clinic presented earlier, the nursing department measured its performance in terms of the number of cases completed in a prescribed time period; satisfaction in the nursing care as indicated by clients, doctors and others; results from client satisfaction surveys; and functioning within budget. Here are some examples of performance indicators that might be developed to demonstrate outcomes for this department:

- the average time when the theatres are not in use: indicator of effective use of facilities.
- the percentage of clients who indicate the nursing care was satisfactory: indicator of client satisfaction.
- the percentage of clients who returned for further surgery/treatment: indicator of satisfactory service.
- the number of staff who remain with the Clinic for more than five years: indicator of staff satisfaction.
- financial statement within budget in one financial year: indicator of financial management.

These indicators measure achievement not activity: relate to objectives: apply only to activities within the control of the staff: are expressed numerically; and are meaningful in terms of the activities of the Clinic.

Common outcomes of the staff development process

Outcomes of the staff development process

1 Introduce new staff to their teams and to their role.
2 Assist the adoption of new roles and responsibilities.
3 Provide continuing learning opportunities.
4 Develop knowledge and skills in processes and procedures.
5 Keep abreast with changing service needs, new knowledge etc.
6 Develop teamwork skills and skills in multi-disciplinary and inter-agency work.
7 Develop methods of evaluating the work in order to learn how to change and improve practice.
8 Provide a structure for effective management of change.
9 Empower individuals to be actively involved in the management of their performance and the organisation.
10 Provide a forum for open communication.

Some of the outcomes identified will occur with specific reference to one or more stages of the process while some will extend over a number of stages. For example, outcomes one and two will likely occur during *orientation* whereas outcomes four and five will likely occur during *continuing education*. Outcomes eight, nine and ten are more generalised and should occur as outcomes of the entire process. These significant overall desirable outcomes will develop over time. Outcomes eight: *effective management of change,* nine: *empowerment,* and ten: *open communication,* warrant further discussion.

Effective management of change

Organisations change all the time if they are dynamic. This continuous change is not necessarily a problem at the organisational level but can be a challenge at the individual level. Change that is self-initiated results in growth and development and usually an improvement in the situation. A conscious decision to change a practice within an organisation is identified as induced change. It can be routine, crisis specific, innovative or transformational. It can arise from the identification of a change in practice, or from client or organisational need. Whatever the nature of change, a general pattern can be identified.

1 There is a need or problem: something is perceived to be not right, or not good enough, or in need of modification or development.
2 There is a period of activity as new ideas are planned, developed and implemented.
3 A change in strategy, people, tactics and/or practice occurs.
4 The organisation settles, people adapt or move on and the organisation survives.

There is a *rational process of change* which if applied, will increase the likelihood of acceptance of the change. This process can be described in stages:

1 **Data are collected to identify the problem or need**
   Data are gathered by survey, documentation, reports, data files, interview, workshop and observation. The problem or need is defined in terms of the scope, how it has been recognised, who is affected, the extent of the situation, what has been tried and what has been successful or has failed.
2 **An assessment and diagnosis of the situation is made**
   The cause(s) of the problem or the need is identified with reference to all variables. At this time caution is advisable in terms of laying blame as single causes are rare. Links within the organisation are identified. The services of a consultant or outside individual can be very useful at this time as those within the organisation may have difficulty viewing the situation objectively; what exists and what is wanted must be clearly identified.
3 **A comprehensive plan is developed**
   This should include objectives, outcomes, indicators, a time frame, an assessment of resources, costing and key players to manage the change. A plan should anticipate responses of individuals which may be fear and the perception of threat, understanding and support, enthusiasm and involvement, rejection and active resistance. Considerable marketing occurs and discussion should be encouraged; the plan may be presented in various drafts for consideration.
4 **The change is implemented according to the plan**
   Careful planning will enhance success and allow for consolidation and stabilisation. Evaluation strategies need to be introduced from the beginning. Management of the transition from old to new becomes an indicator of success and key players are necessary to achieve the outcomes. Achievement is recognised and an environment of support should be fostered.

The most successful change occurs when:

- change is initiated from the top
- a clear set of objectives and a vision are identified
- the change appears sensible to individuals
- timing is appropriate
- effort is put into explaining and selling the benefits
- change is given a high priority
- an understanding exists that change is an ongoing process not a short term solution
- the culture of the organisation is open and innovative.

Change can involve an individual position or a whole department. The need for planned change is equally as important for both.

The staff development process facilitates planned change. In the scenario earlier, the manager identified a change that was needed and went about planning how to implement it. The change was not imposed upon the staff as they were given the opportunity to discuss and question what was planned. An appropriate time was allowed for the new position to develop and outcomes were identified to measure the success of the initiative.

Empowerment

Empowerment is not a new idea. Experiments with self directed work teams have taken place in organisations since the late 1940s. In the last decade global competition has brought about a drive to increase employee participation, commitment and power in the workplace. It is usually a drive for quality that forces the change. Organisations have realised that money does not buy quality, rather that people create quality. Committed people and smart systems are the key although technology does help. Managers can spot quality problems but only employees can prevent problems from happening. This can be seen in health care to a lesser degree than perhaps in business at this stage. Many health care agencies, including hospitals, still have a way to go to realise the importance of the *people they employ*, their staff. A focus on the importance of customer service has helped to create this move towards the empowerment of employees. Only highly skilled, committee empowered employees can be flexible enough to respond quickly to ever changing customer needs.

Perhaps what is new about the idea of empowerment is the strong commitment to self directed work teams by managements who have traditionally resisted employee involvement programs in the past, mainly because such programs have produced changes with which managements have not felt comfortable.

To the individual, empowerment means to give power and authority, to enable and to permit. It implies a notion of self control, direction and result. When people are empowered they adopt an attitude towards their work that passes throughout an entire organisation (Brennan & Horne 1993) and can be seen as:

- full acceptance of accountability
- commitment to an investment in people
- concern to get things done not merely to implement policies
- concern for effective communication
- a positive and genuinely caring attitude to clients, colleagues and themselves
- active, willing participation in management
- commitment to organisational effectiveness because they want to be effective
- a personal code of conduct based on rigorous personal standards and acceptance of responsibility.

Empowerment requires different thinking. It requires people to be prepared to throw away old patterns and behaviours, to accept challenges and to take risks. Empowered behaviour means you are prepared to question what you do, believing there may be a better way. Empowered behaviour will view an unwanted outcome not as a mistake but rather as an opportunity for learning. Empowerment brings about a commitment to learning, gives permission to not always get things right and recognises growth and improvement, no matter how small.

Empowerment often means giving up comfortable practices; giving up something we have done well, received credit for, and feel good about. It often means losing control, at least for an initial period of time and with this comes a loss of security, sometimes mistakes, correction and judgement. But as empowered behaviour within an organisation comes firstly from within the individual and then permeates throughout the organisation, it tends to foster internal growth and cohesion as the organisation takes on the empowered behaviour.

Empowerment in organisations

Unempowered employees	Empowered employees
Are not excited about their work	Feel they make a difference
Feel negative	Are responsible for their results
Don't say what is on their mind	Are part of the team
Only do what they are suppoed to do	Can use their skills and ability
Are suspicious	Control their job
Are not willing to help out	Initiate improvement
Feel they don't matter	Take initiative
Keep their ideas to themselves	Are enthusiastic

The staff development process, because of the relationship it creates between employer and employee, empowers the organisation to grow from its greatest strength, its people. Employees are encouraged to become responsible for their own learning and their own performance. Organisations are realising that their survival depends on the commitment and skills of their staff. During the last decade no significant quality or productivity improvement in a major organisation could have been possible without staff involvement and commitment.

Work with effective leaders in organisations confirms that empowerment requires leadership that creates a sense of ownership of jobs or work by providing clear expectations, controls over resources, responsibility and coaching (Simper & Wilson in Styles 1994). At the heart of organisational empowerment is a belief that the people closest to the work (customer or client) must make the operational decisions. Day to day decisions to achieve competitive levels of quality and service cannot be made in advance or in isolation. Restrictive rules or procedures or inappropriate lines of authority limit decisions. The old way was to define the limits of authority. The new way is to define accountability or measurable results (satisfied customer, quality product) and allow the employee freedom of action to achieve the results. The additional benefit of this approach is that when people feel in charge of their jobs they enjoy them more, and they put more energy into activities that offer them responsibility, respect and identification with outcomes (Simper & Wilson 1993). In other words, they feel empowered.

Health care organisations report similar results when staff are empowered to take control of their jobs and to work towards outcomes that have meaning and relevance. In the scenario earlier, the staff member who was not happy about the new position did not feel able initially to express her concerns but rather imposed her feelings upon the whole group in a negative way. Other members of staff did feel able to express their views and to have input into the planning. After some time and with individual attention and opportunity, the staff member gained confidence and felt more empowered and less threatened by the proposed changes. With the steps that were put into place, staff were able to work towards achieving the outcomes that were meaningful for them. The staff member with the specific concerns gained personal control and increased job satisfaction when given the opportunity to become a clinical teacher.

Open communication

Communication in any day takes many forms: small talk, gossip, critical or sarcastic remarks, commiseration, humour, shop talk, acknowledgment, confidential exchange, compliments, directions, explanation, instruction, and no response.

The concept of open communication is relevant to all situations, and the keys to open communication for individuals are:

- learning to focus on what is being said
- listening attentively
- using appropriate styles
- questioning productively
- remaining open to learning
- avoiding being closed and defensive.

Any staff interaction requires open communication. Within the stages of the staff development process, it is obvious that open communication is crucial. For example:

- If you inquire about a position with the intention of making an application, ask the right questions and listen to what is said about that position.
- If you are in an interview, listen to the words and the intent of the question.
- If you are asking a question, make the purpose clear.
- When someone is talking to you, hold your attention on the speaker rather than letting your mind wander off on an associated thought or in preparation of your answer.

- Say what you mean, not what you think the person wants to hear.
- Allow the speaker to finish; don't interrupt.

Common blocks to open communication include:

- interrupting the speaker
- finishing the sentence for the speaker
- preparing your answer instead of listening
- making assumptions, generalisations and judgements
- failing to attend; that is, with body posture, reflection, or acknowledgment
- using closed questions
- defending your position and views rather than appreciating the point of view of another.

Communication on an organisational level is based upon the same principles. For a staff development manager or staff development co-ordinator, the following principles apply (Donovan & Jackson 1992):

Enhancing managerial communication

Open up communication channels throughout the organisation
Plan formal communication
Orient the message to the receiver's experiences
Be aware of non-verbal cues that enhance meaning
Respond to feedback
Strive for clarity of message content
Keep language simple and suitable to the audience
Be aware of the importance of timing
Recognise that the process of communication is often of greater importance than the message transmitted
Recognise that what you do may be more important than what you say
Avoid unnecessary meetings
Follow up formal communication to determine if the intended action was taken
Regulate information flow
Encourage mutual trust
Use the informal communication network where necessary and appropriate.

In the scenario earlier, open communication assisted the nurse to identify her concerns in the interview that the manager held with the nurse who felt unhappy about the new planned position. The manager listened and reflected on what was said and then tried to understand what the nurse was saying both with words and feelings. The importance of open communication has also been described earlier in this book in terms of its importance to learning and teaching.

Chapter summary

The staff development process is a series of sequential stages that link together as part of a process of learning and development. The staff development process is equally as important to the employer as it is to the employee. However, for it to be successful both employer and employee must perceive benefits from the investment of resources into the development of the process. The integration of the staff development process within total management of the organisation has been presented in this chapter with a work place scenario, where each stage of the process was described and demonstrated by an actual experience. The application of performance appraisal as the tool for performance management was then described with examples of performance indicators from the previous work place scenario. Finally, common outcomes of a staff development process were given as effective management of change, empowerment and open communication.

REFERENCES

Brennan B, Horner B 1993 Empowerment and total health care employee involvement: the first steps to high performance with high commitment. IES Conferences Australia, NSW

Donovan F, Jackson A C 1991 Managing human service organisations. Prentice Hall Sydney

Guinn K 1990 Performance management: not just annual appraisal. Training and Development Journal October: 39-45

Mayo T 1992 Performance indicators for community organisation. Council of Social Services of New South Wales, Allans, Surrey Hills

Styles M M 1994 International Nursing Review 41(3):77-80

5

Options for staff development

Key questions

- How does an organisation establish a commitment to staff development?

- How does an organisation manage a staff development process?

- Should staff development be centralised or decentralised?

- How can the staff development process be implemented throughout the organisation?

- What are the advantages and disadvantages of mandatory and voluntary staff education?

- How can you demonstrate financial accountability for staff development?

Content summary

Introduction

The establishment of a staff development process occurs when an organisation is committed to staff development and committed to a learning environment. The process can be managed in different ways and can be implemented using different strategies. This Chapter will first describe how an organisation can create a learning environment within an organisation. It will then describe a centralised and decentralised way to manage the staff development process. Different implementation approaches will be described as well as the use of both internal and external resources. Finally, the issue of financial accountability for staff development will be discussed.

Establishing a commitment to staff development

Staff development is a term familiar to most health care organisations but is usually used in reference to education and training activities. In nursing, staff development was designated as a stream within the career structure of the 1980s and nurses were employed in *Staff Development* positions. A staff development position meant that some component of the role, usually clinical teaching and perhaps some other formal teaching responsibilities, was designated to staff development functions.

In nursing in the 1990s, it is more common to see the position *Clinical Nurse Specialist*. The position includes among other things a responsibility for supervising, teaching and appraising staff in the clinical area. This does not usually include budget responsibilities but may include other personnel functions. Designated *Staff Development* positions are far less common. There is usually a management position, a *Nurse Manager* as well as a Clinical Nurse Specialist, where the manager has responsibility for running the unit with all the usual management responsibilities. In nursing today the situation has been further modified with a *Clinical Manager* position that appears to be a mixture of all of the above responsibilities, designed to combine both a staff development and management role.

I do not believe that any of the above situations necessarily demonstrates a commitment to the development of staff and certainly does not demonstrate a staff development process. At best it may indicate allocation of resources to the orientation of new staff and to clinical teaching when it is needed. At worst it indicates role confusion and unrealistic expectations of performance of the individuals who hold the multi-role positions. It represents a minimal or beginning commitment to the development of staff.

A health care organisation with a commitment to the development of staff would demonstrate a corporate or executive position with clear accountability for monitoring and developing the human resources of the organisation. In addition, the organisation would have devolved responsibility for the development of staff to a division or department, rather than at a corporate level of control. The organisation's investment in staff and their expectations of staff would be clearly articulated and each individual employee would be expected to show a commitment through their performance. It is not the number of people who are allocated, the presence or lack of presence of a staff development department, nor the size of the budget that makes the difference. It is the culture and commitment of the entire organisation.

How can this be achieved? First, management should take the lead in demonstrating that staff development is essential to the organisation's effective and efficient functioning, and second, the organisation should demonstrate a commitment to learning.

Management view of staff development

The benefits of staff development are not self evident. Staff development is often seen as a discretionary expense and not an essential component of the business. It is not in the same league in the corporate mind as marketing or finance or operations divisions. Employers through managers may admit that training is necessary at times, but they do not always recognise that training is only one component of staff development.

Managers may say in all honesty that people are their most important resource and may think they are making a commitment through training, but when it comes to the (economic) crunch, expenses are inevitably cut in areas involving staff development. Those aspects of the staff development process seen to be within routine personnel functions are likely to be accepted as necessary, but the value of an overall process is often not seen. Managers often expect staff development to fix problems: to increase skills, to stretch resources that are available, to deal with a difficult staff member or one not performing to expectation, to address staff concerns, or to keep staff happy.

When it comes to estimating the value an organisation places on its employees, the staff development budget is a useful indicator. Analysts would look for a commitment of finance to staff development before believing that an organisation really considered it was important. Such expenditure might be seen in a number of areas, such as:

- money allocated for all staff to attend conferences and seminars, regardless of level of seniority
- money allocated to computer training and updates
- occupational health and safety and ergonomic monitoring and education
- money to purchase educational materials and resources
- two or three days allocated to the orientation of new staff

- performance requirements within a job description to show a commitment to ongoing learning
- time allocated to compulsory attendance at on-the-job education sessions, usually held at the end of a shift.

Less common areas might include:

- budget to allow new staff to work as supernumerary for the first two weeks
- time allocated for all staff to attend education sessions
- money allocated to a variety of learning facilities and resources
- budget allocated to allow for departmental strategic planning sessions
- release of staff for time out, de-briefing sessions or stress related recovery
- budget for social functions to build teams and create opportunities for networking and interaction.

A long term study conducted by a training magazine over a period of seven years asked organisations to classify expenditure into five categories (Lee 1988a). Over years the categories for the classification of expenditure varied, but the following list was the most comprehensive. It had attempted to identify all expenditure:

1 Hardware: computers, audiovisual and video equipment

2 Off the shelf materials: books, films, computer software, class room courses and selection tools

3 Custom materials: audio visual material, videos, printed material, computer courses and staff profiling packages

4 Seminars, conferences etc: training provided by outside providers on or off the premises

5 Outside services: fees for consultants not acting in a training role

6 Training staff salaries and organisation overheads.

Analysis of data collected from some 100 organisations indicated that formal training budgets, as designated by the above list, account for only about 70% of the organisations' actual training purchases. In other words training expenses incurred by other departments that never appear in a formal training budget might well add another 30% to the average organisations' training account. The point the study was making from this was to demonstrate how difficult it was to calculate meaningful figures for training expenditure.

Such common categories are necessary for resource accountability but again do not necessarily indicate an overall commitment. The following is a list of uncommon but advantageous strategies that an organisation might consider. Each of them would indicate a more convincing commitment to the development of staff and they are not all expensive. Take the time to examine your organisation and identify if any of them are present.

A commitment to staff development

- A clear statement of the organisation's mission and philosophy given to every new staff member upon employment and to every staff member on their anniversary date (or at Christmas). The mission statement includes a commitment to staff and their importance in the attainment of the organisation's goals.
- A statement about the importance of people placed within every department, easily visible to staff and clients.
- Time allocated in every orientation program for new staff to hear and discuss the organisation's mission, philosophy and goals presented by senior staff.
- Resources allocated for strategic planning sessions with all staff or appropriate representation of staff (selected by the staff) from all areas and departments, making sure that all levels of staff have the opportunity to participate.
- Recognition given to education for skills, knowledge and personal development as identified by either the staff member or the manager, or both, regardless of how unusual it may seem.
- Regular recognition of staff achievement and/or commitment through a staff newsletter, informal award or simply a letter.
- An annual organisation-wide staff needs assessment.
- Innovative advertisements for positions that encourage people to apply and to show initiative.
- The use of multiple strategies to collect information for staff selection that might include job resumes, interviews, organisation initiated referee contact, case studies, human resource assessment testing techniques; to demonstrate that the organisation is looking for the best person for the job, not the one who is available at the time.
- An ongoing self appraisal system where staff, peers and managers give and receive regular informal feedback, combined with a structured annual review based on goal setting and forward planning .
- Opportunities for open discussion upon cessation of employment.
- A corporate structure that includes an executive position who functions as an adviser and resource *not* as a manager, with responsibility for coordinating the staff development initiatives of the organisation.

How many strategies like these exist in your organisation? In what ways do you see your organisation's commitment to staff development? What management behaviours are evident? In an organisation which can demonstrate a commitment to staff development, such behaviours will be evident in every individual throughout the organisation but *must* be evident at the management level if the process is to be real.

Donovan and Jackson (1991) propose seven core competencies required by public service managers. Public service managers have similar roles to health service managers and both hold responsibility for the management of their human resources. The core competencies identified for public service managers are equally as applicable for health service managers. The core competencies identified could be viewed as evidence of a commitment by management personnel to staff development. The organisation should determine the strategies to achieve the competencies in each area of management. The seven competencies are as follows:

- manage people: demonstrate the ability to lead with vision, communicate clearly, manage team performance and manage conflict and negotiation
- determine client service: demonstrate the ability to set standards, research needs and improve services
- act strategically: demonstrate the ability to respond politically and to manage stakeholders
- achieve results: demonstrate the ability to plan, control and organise; add value to products and services; accept responsibility
- create solutions: demonstrate the ability to make decisions and solve problems
- act entrepreneurially: demonstrate the ability to manage change and complexity, to create options
- continue self development: demonstrate the ability to assess needs and initiate self development.

Creating a learning organisation

A learning organisation is one where the people all work together striving to achieve common goals, with an open mind to change (Sofo 1993). In health care organisations, the learners are mainly adult learners and so the principles of adult learning have relevance to the concept of a learning health care organisation. The principles of adult learning, commonly associated with Malcolm Knowles, can be applied to health care organisations. People as a group within an organisation need to know why they need to learn. People as a group within an organisation need to feel like an autonomous group or entity and have a sense of being self-directing with the ability to build on their shared experiences and skills. As a group or empowered team they recognise a total group readiness and are sensitive to learning in relation to real work/life issues. People acting as an entity will wish to achieve the best results because they will be a better organisation, able to build on their own development and common experiences.

The result of an organisation committed to learning is a realisation that the outcomes are greater than any of the individuals, or the sum of the individuals. As in an orchestra, where the sound of a symphony is far richer than the sound of each individual instrument or the instruments playing together, the impact of the outcomes of an organisation committed to learning, are as rich for the organisation as they are for each individual. While learning occurs in many settings, for many adults about 50% of all learning is work related. Work itself can be learning, where individuals equate work to learning new things all the time. When individuals learn, organisations learn; and when they learn they can adapt their behaviour on the basis of past experiences and skills as well as invent new behaviours and practices. The organisation remains open and aware and ready to change. An organisation with a commitment to learning has the following characteristics (Dixon 1992):

Demonstration of an organisational commitment to learning

- There is a holistic view of the organisation where departments are viewed as equally important; common vision is evident in the way people behave; resources are shared and exchanged; people move freely between departments.
- The organisation obtains and uses information about the external environment; it has an awareness of the whole community (health care system); it has knowledge of other agencies with whom it interacts; it collaborates with other agencies.
- The organisation develops new knowledge; creates an opportunity for innovative research; seeks out opportunities for development.
- The organisation learns from alliances with other organisations; this entails prior agreement on responsibilities, objectives and effective communication.
- The organisation retrieves and retains organisational memory; information is disseminated throughout the organisation.
- The organisation clarifies and communicates success and failure; colleagues are open and honest in their opinions and seek assurance that communication will be respectful and discreet.
- There is direct feedback on performance; regular meetings provide a forum for open discussion.
- The organisation questions assumptions; maintains a productive and innovative self awareness.
- The organisation coaches individuals using the method as a shared problem solving approach; communicates respect; is change oriented and disciplined.

As with individuals, organisations need to be open to new ideas and to view them as opportunities for growth and learning. Organisations which are closed to new ideas tend to present as protective, threatened and defensive and it is unlikely that learning will take place in this environment. A learning organisation is an organisation that facilitates the learning of all its members and continuously transforms itself (Pedler et al 1991).

The metaphor of the learning organisation is a powerful one. It treats the organisation as a personified organism with the ability to adapt to changing environments. The organisation's identity has the ability to be more than the sum of the individuals and new shared strength and knowledge will improve the performance of the whole organisation. There are two essential elements to the notion of a learning organisation. First, that the group (organisational) goals are attained and second, that shared responsiveness is critical to such attainment. Dixon (1992) speaks of two types of learning essential to excellent organisations: innovative learning and adaptive learning. Organisations can act as well as adapt in a similar way to people, that is, reactively or proactively to their environments. When organisations learn, they adapt their behaviour on the basis of past experiences and skills as well as invent new behaviours and try new skills, to anticipate obstacles to their goal achievement.

An organisation that is open to learning will create a culture where individuals are recognised and facilitated to develop to their potential. Individuals will feel rewarded and, therefore, committed to the goals of the organisation. The staff development process provides the framework upon which such commitment can be developed and demonstrated. Learning of any sort can only occur within a supportive environment.

Managing the staff development process

A discussion about management, be it the management of training, human resources or personnel responsibilities, will inevitably lead towards a discussion about the merits of centralisation or decentralisation. Perhaps the most important consideration to keep in mind has been best summarised by Tom Humphrey, chairman and CEO of the Forum Corporation in Boston, USA, who commented:

Does a company see training as a key element in creating its competitive advantage? If it does, training will be in close proximity to the core activities of the business. If it doesn't, it will screw around with [the question of] whether training should be centralised or decentralised (Lee 1988b).

It does not have to be a matter of either/or as there is a place for both management styles in any one organisation at any one time. What is important is that the organisation allows itself to evolve into what is best for the organisation. At the moment within the health care system the trend is towards decentralisation of management practices thanks to corporate staff slashing, increasingly advanced technology and a desire to stay attuned to the customer mentality.

Organisations are, however, decentralising practices without appropriate consideration of either the process or the outcomes. What often happens is that the system appears on paper to be decentralised. In terms of its functioning however, it remains in the control of a central management system.

The merits of a *decentralised* staff development function can be identified as:

- greater immediacy of response
- credibility and a sense of ownership
- cost effectiveness
- less complex systems.

The failings of a *decentralised* staff development function can, however, counteract these. They are:

- inconsistency
- poor quality due to a lack of centralised standards
- assumed capability of providers
- difficulty with accountability.

It is useful to view the options along a continuum of control where it is recognised that some functions are better centralised and some better decentralised. Centralisation can provide some safeguards for the organisation. For example:

- A corporate culture can be established and maintained.
- Leadership can be demonstrated and viewed.
- The organisation can present a clear vision and mission.
- A customer/client focus can be established.
- Rationalisation of resources can occur.
- Common functions and activities can be implemented.

Some activities lend themselves to centralisation, particularly in the personnel area of responsibility. An organisation may purchase common resources for departments at a more cost effective rate. Organisation-wide contracts can be negotiated for consultancy services, information technology training and updates. A corporate workshop or residential program could be negotiated at a much more cost effective rate than if it were negotiated by numerous departments. A centralised advisory and resource department could be of great value to the organisation and to individual managers. If an organisation is considering decentralisation it is useful to examine the reasons behind the consideration. Ask the question, what is behind this decision? The following questions may guide a useful inquiry:

- Does the decision reflect economic (staff) cutbacks rather than consideration of what is good for the organisation?
- Where will the accountability and control be for those functions that have been decentralised?
- Are managers just being asked to do more with less resources?
- Who will be accountable, what outcomes will be measured and by whom?
- How has the budget been allocated to account for the activities that have been decentralised?
- Whose needs are really being met?

There are certainly aspects of the staff development process that could be centralised to achieve better outcomes, greater satisfaction and consistency.

Centralised staff development functions

- Development of advertisements for positions to portray the corporate image
- Selection processes and procedures
- Negotiation of work place agreements and contracts
- Corporate orientation
- Provision of continuing education resources
- Negotiations with outside consultants for organisation-wide activities
- Development of guidelines for promotion and recognition
- Development of organisation mechanisms for feedback including performance appraisal tools
- Information technology training
- Organisation wide research

Decentralised staff development functions

- Budget allocation and responsibility for staff education and development
- Management of human resources including, selection, appointment, • promotion, appraisal and exit
- Orientation of staff to a position and department
- Continuing education initiatives
- Staff needs assessment
- Local research initiatives
- Ongoing performance appraisal

When determining centralisation or decentralisation, it is important that an organisation consider its overall management plan taking into account the organisation's culture, characteristics, qualities (qualifications) and short–comings. Decisions should not be made in isolation. The management plan needs to be consistent but does not have to be exactly the same in all key areas of functioning. In summary, decisions about centralisation/decentralisation should consider all factors, not only cost effectiveness. An organisation will grow towards decentralisation as it matures and develops, as will the individuals within it.

Mandatory v. voluntary staff development

An organisation functions in respect of its structures, procedures, personnel, external influences, outcomes and economic and political influences. We all know of organisations that seem to just *keep on keeping on,* without being able to identify any specific reason or explanation for their consistent performance. Individuals come to work, do their job and produce results. Nothing really good seems to happen; but neither does anything of significant concern. Individuals do not appear to initiate growth and development, neither does the organisation impose growth upon the individual. Certainly an organisation can survive in this manner but it will not attain a competitive edge. Individuals within the organisation will not achieve their potential, nor will they attain a high level of job satisfaction.

If the organisation wants growth to occur, it will need to introduce an incentive to learn within the organisation. You cannot *make* people grow but you can facilitate their growth. The organisation must determine the nature of the incentive it wishes to introduce. At one end of the continuum they may involve compulsory activities while at the other they may involve voluntary activities. It is useful to consider the debate regarding mandatory or voluntary staff development.

The debate usually occurs in respect of continuing education; should health professionals have to attend continuing education to maintain practice standards, or should they be able to decide according to need. The debate around the two options does have application to all stages of the staff development process. The following examples show how the issue of mandatory versus compulsory staff development has application through all the stages of the staff development process:

Stage: recruitment, selection and appointment
Issue: does the organisation require that all those involved in selection of staff attend a course on selection techniques, or do they rely upon individual knowledge and expertise?
Stage: orientation and consolidation
Issue: is time spent attending orientation sessions compulsory and recorded as part of performance appraisal, regardless of previous experience?
Stage: continuing education
Issue: does the organisation require that every staff member attend a certain number and nature of seminars and workshops during the year of employment, or are they allowed to choose their own?
Stage: promotion and exit
Issue: are promotional appointments made only when evidence of continuing learning can be demonstrated, which might include pursuit of further studies and qualifications?

In terms of continuing education, staff learn to:

• gain knowledge, skills and attitudes that will enable the individual to perform better
• develop competence in a new role, in a new technique or in acquiring a behaviour
• enhance self development and personal growth

An organisation learns to:

- expand services
- improve performance
- increase customer satisfaction.

In health care, the overall goal of learning is to improve health care through changed practices. In nursing, the primary objective in continuing learning is the improvement of professional practice to meet the needs of the client population. Learning can be identified as having occurred when there is a change in the individual caused by the interaction of that individual with the environment, which fills a need, improves the ability to deal with some aspect of the environment and leads to the acquisition of new behaviours. An organisation will aim to bring about a *change in the individual* to meet the needs of the organisation, through a process of learning. For the individual, the learning may be directed toward:

- attaining a specific goal (make something happen)
- performing a specific activity (acquire a new skill)
- acquiring new information (learning for learning's sake).

Determining if staff development is to be mandatory or voluntary will not necessarily upgrade or improve performance and service. The decision is only the beginning of the process for neither will make people learn.

The desire for continuing learning is a life long commitment and is part of an individual's total behaviour and cannot be guaranteed regardless of whether the learning is made mandatory or voluntary. Continuing learning is an essential part of performance, a tool to be used to achieve a required/desired outcome. Learning through staff development at best promotes competence and knowledge, and at the very least exposes individuals to information that they would otherwise not encounter. However, the decision to learn is made by the individual regardless of the structures that are imposed. Unfortunately, the assumption is made that if learning is made compulsory, it will happen. As has been discussed in Chapter 3, this is not necessarily the case. It is useful to review some of the characteristics of mandatory and voluntary staff development.

Mandatory staff development

- Forces attendance but does not ensure competence
- Discourages self initiated or self directed learning
- Often occurs after the failure of a voluntary system
- Creates negative and resentful attitudes
- Tends to encourage individuals to learn to play the system
- Disempowers the individual

Voluntary staff development

- Encourages self assessment of ability
- Excludes those most likely to need learning who are least likely to be involved
- Individuals are more likely to choose to learn
- Learning relates to need and therefore has more relevance
- Encourages responsibility and accountability
- Empowers the individual

An organisation must make a decision as to what is best for that organisation and the individuals within it. If continuing education is considered by the organisation to be part of a commitment to continuing learning, the following statement is worthy of note. *Participation in continuing education does not generate competence, but not having to (participate), guarantees even less* (Lowenthal 1988).

Implementing the staff development process

Having determined a commitment to staff development, created a learning environment within the organisation and established a management approach that supports a commitment to staff development, it is time to consider how to implement the process. Again, because most resources are allocated to the orientation-consolidation-continuing education stages of the process, much of the discussion about implementation relates to those stages. The principles can still be applied to all stages.

Approaches to implementation

Three approaches are presented here:

- structured approach
- semi-structured approach
- self-directed approach

A *structured approach* tends towards a centralised model of management where most activities are compulsory. Staff are given little choice, programs are set well in advance and repeated, routines are followed and techniques remain the same. Practices are predictable, consistent and not necessarily based on individual need. There is a great deal of value to be gained from a structured approach and some components of the staff development process particularly lend themselves to structure; for example, recruitment, selection and appointment. Characteristics include:

- effective use of resources
- cost effectiveness
- consistency
- credibility if well evaluated
- standardisation.

Within a structured approach you would expect to see some or all of the following:

Characteristics of structured activities

- Standard advertisements and job descriptions
- Common selection processes used throughout the organisation
- Standard letters and conditions of employment
- A centralised corporate organisation-wide orientation and consolidation program
- A well planned and ordered program of continuing education with little choice, planned for the whole year
- Predictable promotional appointments
- Routine exit questionnaire and interview
- Little evidence of initiative and creativity
- A sense of routine and predicability within the organisation
- Staff designated with responsibility for staff development

A *semi-structured approach* has many similar characteristics to the structured approach. However it does allow for a more needs based approach to staff development and accommodates more flexibility and initiative. Characteristics include:

- guidelines for the effective use or resources but flexibility allowed
- more cost effective if monitored carefully
- some consistency but also considerable flexibility
- credibility if well evaluated
- standardisation of outcomes.

Within a semi-structured approach you would expect to see some of the following characteristics but not necessarily all.

Characteristics of semi-structured activities

- Standard advertisements and job descriptions
- Common selection processes used throughout the organisation
- Standard letters and conditions of employment
- A centralised corporate organisation-wide orientation program, as well as decentralised departmental orientation and consolidation programs
- A well planned and ordered program for continuing education with a range of options for development according to need
- Predictable promotional opportunities but the opportunity for individual nomination and initiative
- Routine exit questionnaire and interview
- Much more opportunity for initiative and creativity
- A sense of routine and predictability combined with a sense of initiative
- Staff designated with responsibility for staff development

A *self-directed approach* is likely to be implemented only within the orientation-consolidation-continuing education stages, with either of the other approaches applying to the other stages. A self-directed approach has particular characteristics:

- a variety of resources with some consistency but considerable variation
- expensive especially in the development stage
- difficult to evaluate consistently as value relates to individual need
- principles may still be standardised.

Within a self-directed approach you would expect to see all or some of the following:

Characteristics of self-directed activities

- Standard advertisements and job descriptions
- Common selection processes used throughout the organisation
- Standard letters and conditions of employment
- Needs-based orientation and consolidation programs
- Guidelines for expected or core continuing education programs plus the opportunity for self-selection in areas of need and interest; a department may establish a *credit point system* and allow staff to select options in accordance with the total credits allocated (for example, out of a total of 50 credits for the year, a conference = 10 credits, an approved learning package = 5 credits)
- Greater likelihood of self initiated promotional advancement based on individual merit and initiative
- Routine exit questionnaire and interview, perhaps conducted less formally
- Considerable evidence of initiative and creativity
- A sense of opportunity, initiative and fairness while maintaining some predicability
- Departmental managers will usually have designated responsibility for staff development

It is likely that an organisation will show evidence of all three approaches to implementation with variation between departments and/or professional groups. When choosing an approach, organisations should be mindful of a number of factors including:

- budget constraints
- staff expertise
- staff availability and flexibility
- nature of the work force; that is, the number of people in positions and the number of different positions
- management model(s) within the organisation
- resources and facilities

- client characteristics and needs
- services offered
- economic and political constraints.

Again the most appropriate approach will depend on a number of factors including the stage of development of the organisation. An organisation may choose different approaches according to its stage of growth.

Implementation using internal resources

With this approach the organisation must have access to expertise, resources and facilities within the organisation. There may be an organisation-wide *staff development department*, with a manager (co-ordinator) and staff appointed for their qualifications and experience, possibly allocated to divisions or departments. There may be *a corporate adviser* appointment who acts as a resource for staff appointed to a department/division, where the process is being implemented. Specifically, the organisation will need:

- facilities and space for teaching and learning activities
- audiovisual resources for teaching such as overhead projectors, slides, and sound system
- staff with appropriate qualifications and expertise
- clinical experts
- mentors and/or preceptors
- an administrative structure to support the programs
- clearly defined programs.

A staff development program may be designed to have *core components* for all staff, for departments/divisions and *optional components* that are position specific, or seniority specific. Examples of all of these are given below:

Organisation-wide core components

- Occupational health and safety principles and practices
- Corporate culture, mission and goals
- Structure and function of the organisation
- Performance management systems and processes
- Health care organisation systems
- Customer/client focus principles and practices

Departmental/division core components

- Client services (for example, within the nursing division)
- Clinical knowledge, skills (for example, within the nursing division)
- Catering services (for example, clerical staff, administrative support services)
- Profession specific topics (for example, legal accountability for nursing)

111

Position-specific components: manager

- Selection processes and strategies
- Team building
- Leadership
- Peer appraisal
- Budgeting
- Case management
- Negotiation
- Problem solving and decision making

This approach usually includes on-the-job staff development, meaning that staff development activities occur while the individual is working, rather than releasing the individual from work. Such practices are sometimes perceived to be simple and fast; it is thought that they require little planning and that anyone can do it. This is not necessarily the case. There are certain considerations to ensure that this type of staff development is successful:

1 Pre-planning is necessary to identify skills, performance standards, demonstration techniques, evaluation methods, time and resource allocation.
2 Staff in a preceptor role should be selected carefully: as they are required to demonstrate, they should have expertise and be willing and available.
3 Support materials should be available, such as manuals, handbooks and examples of documentation to reinforce learning.
4 Time should be allocated to ensure that teaching and learning is productive.
5 Ongoing and formative evaluation is an essential component and strategies should be established before learning begins.
6 Learning should be based on need: a thorough assessment of current level of knowledge and expertise should be conducted before the learning occurs.

There is a great deal to be gained by an approach that uses internal resources. However, it is resource intensive and does require significant administrative infrastructure.

Implementation using external resources

This approach allows the organisation to utilise other resources as well as their own. An organisation may choose to do this for a number of reasons, such as lack of facilities, insufficient resources (equipment), lack of staff expertise in a particular area, insufficient staff numbers to accommodate release of staff, inappropriate administrative infrastructure, or better quality (value) resources available elsewhere. The structure of a program may still include organisation-wide, departmental/division and/or position core components and the content of each could be the same as was suggested for implementation using internal resources. It is likely that the responsibility for staff development will be more decentralised throughout the organisation with this approach, as there is more of a facilitator/organiser/co-ordinator role most of the time. It would be advantageous to have an organisation resource/adviser role with this approach to facilitate access to information and resources. This approach allows for access to a number of options.

Consultants

The role of the consultant has become attractive to many individuals who feel they have specific marketable knowledge and expertise, resources for independent practice, or who have become disillusioned working as an employee and seek to be their own boss. Consultants can be found in all areas of staff development as they can be in other areas. A consultant may be approached to present information; to work within an organisation in a specific area of expertise for a period of time; to review, evaluate and report on practices; or to conduct a staff development activity. Consultants sell their expertise often using glossy documents and brochures, reports from past jobs or other promotional material. It is easy to be overpowered by a consultant especially if the organisation is keen to engage someone to solve a problem. Always remember, you are the one purchasing, so do your homework and check the consultant out in the same way you check out an employee or new product. Make sure the consultant is prepared to meet your needs and is not trying to fit you into a standard model, or liken you to other customers. Don't be influenced by their price, slick presentation or list of satisfied customers. A consultant should be able to:

- provide evidence of qualifications in the area for which they are being consulted
- provide evidence of experience working with similar organisations
- be prepared to come to the organisation to discuss and to work
- be prepared to listen to your needs rather than propose a solution
- adapt their work to the characteristics and needs of the organisation
- demonstrate a competitive fee structure
- provide routine follow up on their work and seek out evaluation.

Seminars, conferences, workshops

The volume of literature that comes to the desk of anyone involved in staff development is amazing. Providers spend huge amounts of money producing glossy brochures designed to convince you that you must attend a seminar, or cannot afford to miss out on an opportunity. The language is persuasive, the benefits are thrust upon you, and the value for money is fiercely proclaimed. In health care there seems to be an abundance of conferences, while in training and management there appears to be an abundance of seminars. How can you possibly determine what is valuable? How can you decide between them all? The decision to attend, or to send a staff member to a seminar, conference or workshop should be based upon the specific need at the time, giving consideration to preferred learning style, and current state of awareness/desire

113

for information. Other more pragmatic factors such as budget, employer preference, and support that is available should also be considered. There is a place for conferences, seminars and workshops but they are all slightly different.

Conferences

- Usually one to three days in length
- Target professional groups, organisations and associations in a particular field; for example, human resource managers, clinical nursing, continuing education providers, health service executives
- Speakers should be chosen for knowledge, experience, and presentation ability (although the latter is often forgotten)
- Material should provide something for everyone, be well balanced and state of the art
- Provide an excellent opportunity for networking and interacting
- Provide an opportunity to increase knowledge and skills, although learning is not necessarily immediately applicable to the work place.

Seminars

- Usually one day; occasionally extends to two days
- Numbers often very large
- Target almost anyone on any particular topic, although material usually identifies particular groups; for example, senior managers, leaders, specific qualifications
- Speakers are often pre-selected by the provider because of presentation skills, not just their knowledge and expertise
- Material is general and sometimes superficial
- Little opportunity for networking and interaction as the program is usually fully structured and the presentation dominates
- Provide an opportunity to increase knowledge and skills, and, learning may be able to be applied directly to the work place.

Workshops

- Usually one day; occasionally residential
- Target specific groups; numbers usually restricted; for example, peri–operative nurses with 60 places
- Facilitator (not lecturer or speaker) should have knowledge and considerable expertise in the area and as a facilitator
- Material should be specific, relevant and immediately useable
- Material should be presented to facilitate interaction and participation
- Excellent opportunity for networking and peer learning/support
- Provide an opportunity to increase knowledge and skill (professional and personal) and learning should be directly applicable to the individual's situation (professional or personal).

Other providers

It is possible to negotiate with another agency, educational institution or agency to give access to resources, either on an informal or formal basis. Informally, it may involve making information available to staff, purchasing existing material for staff to utilise, reserving regular places in courses for staff, and negotiating to contribute financially towards costs for staff. Here are some examples of such arrangements that exist in the market today:

- Promotional material from a provider is distributed throughout the organisation and the provider offers a discount price for staff individually or in a group.
- The agency regularly hires educational videos for circulation throughout the organisation.
- The organisation purchases a self-directed learning package on a topic for staff to work through in their own time.
- The organisation negotiates to have the provider reserve a number of places in course and always sends staff.
- The organisation negotiates with staff to pay a percentage of a fee for an existing course or seminar.

More formal arrangements may also occur:

- An organisation may contract a provider to conduct a training needs assessment and then to develop an organisation-wide staff development program.
- Two organisations in a region may contract to share the expense of hiring a provider to present or develop a program.
- An organisation may contract with a tertiary institution to enrol staff into a course; for example, a *Certificate in Aged Care*.
- An organisation may contract with another organisation to have staff work with that organisation for a period of time to gain experience in a particular area. This could be a two-way arrangement.
- An organisation may contract a company to conduct all staff recruitment and selection.

The possibilities are endless if an organisation is prepared to be innovative. Many organisations would welcome an opportunity to share resources, facilities and/or expertise.

Financial accountability

Of all the areas of responsibility of a management role within human service organisations, it is the control of financial matters and budgeting that appears to cause most concern. Why is this so? First, there is a common perception that if you are concerned with the health (well being, welfare) of a client group and with bringing about good outcomes, then concern about finances and costing seems to be in conflict with service delivery and meeting needs.

Second, management of budgets and finances is perceived as a technical component of the role and outside the usual expertise of a human service manager.

The reality is that staff development must be budgeted and accounted for in an acceptable manner. One of the major problems in human service organisations and therefore in health care organisations like hospitals, is the existence of a 'them and us' mentality.

The financial side of the organisation sees the service providers as unrealistic spenders who need to be controlled, where the service providers see the finance side as 'bean counters' obsessed with cost cutting.

The difficulty of demonstrating measurable (quantitative) outcomes from staff development initiatives has been referred to earlier. How do you demonstrate that someone has learnt something that will improve service delivery? How can you know that a selection assessment program will ensure that the best candidate is employed and that the organisation will benefit? How do you demonstrate long term value to the organisation of sending twenty managers to a two day residential strategic planning workshop? It is an error to attempt to argue the merits (value) of an intended or actual program on a cost saving basis.

It is also unwise to claim future savings from current expenditure in an area without supportive data. It is difficult to place a monetary value on a staff development activity often because outcomes of activities cannot be measured at the time; because activities are not necessarily of equal value; because activities vary in their ability to achieve outcomes. Have you heard this said: *We are all sitting around here at this seminar and it is costing $$$ in salary alone, when we could be working.* The cost of the seminar can only be considered if it can be compared to an activity of equal value, which has been sacrificed for the seminar. Or if the seminar was considered a waste of time. Unfortunately, referring to something as *a cost* often gives rise to a negative value.

Vinter and Kish in Donovan and Jackson (1991) suggest that budgeting and programming activities have become separated in most human service organisations. As a result they are often competing.

Budgeting and programming—conditions giving rise to perceived differences

- Division of labour and structures within agencies results in separate units with different personnel working in each of them, where neither unit really understands the value of the other.
- Necessary career specialisation in each area exacerbates the perceived differences
- Differences in daily routines makes their work appear different.
- Economic decisions of the organisation place the two areas against each other, with programmers feeling they are victims of financial decisions.

- Senior level management perpetuate the differences with a lack of understanding.

A useful way to demonstrate the value of staff development initiatives can be through a *cost effective analysis*. If the organisation has a commitment to staff development and it is a learning organisation, a well presented cost effective analysis is probably the most useful way to present all the data that is available so that value can be evaluated. It must be remembered, however, that budgeting is an overall organisation concern and all staff development activities need to be considered within the context of the overall budget. There are often other factors, not necessarily identified, that may influence the result.

Cost-effective analysis: steps for development

1 Identify the objective to be achieved for the specific target group.
2 Specify optimal programs to be used.
3 Determine costs for each program, cost per unit of service and amount of service rendered.
4 Assess the effect of the outcome of the program on the target group.
5 Combine the cost and the outcome information to present a cost outcome and cost effectiveness analyses.

Some simple guidelines for demonstrating value from staff development are:

- Be realistic in your evaluation.
- Identify needs and relate to the program of choice.
- State clear objectives and realistic outcomes.
- Identify short term and long term benefits.
- Present qualitative measures as well as quantitative measures.
- Present evaluation strategies.
- Be prepared to give and take.

The following examples demonstrate how value can be demonstrated:

Example

The demand for expertise in a specific clinical skill has increased. You identify a small number of staff to be given the opportunity to develop skills in the area. Calculate the cost to include the cost of education plus the cost to replace them while they are away. Identify the number of times the expertise in this area has been requiredand the cost to bring someone in from another area to provide that expertise. Demonstrate how developing expertise within this small group can be taught to other staff members over time.

Example

An international conference in Palliative Care is advertised and three staff identify that they would like to attend. The cost is significant and involves travel to another capital city. If these staff attend, the unit will be without some senior staff for the time they will be away. Calculate the total cost of sending three staff, recognising that if they all attend, the combined knowledge will be of considerable use to the unit. Invite the staff concerned to identify how they plan to utilise the knowledge they will obtain at the conference when they return, for themselves and for the unit. Ask them to prepare a combined staff development program. Demonstrate that the new knowledge and expertise will expand the services of the unit and will increase the range of services that can be offered. Demonstrate how the skills that they will bring back can be 'bought' by other units both within the hospital and elsewhere.

Chapter summary

This chapter has examined two key concepts that contribute to the success of a staff development process; management's view of staff development and the creation of a learning environment within the organisation. The view of management will determine the overall commitment to staff development and the creation of a learning environment will mean that the organisation is open to change and to development. Having established this commitment, the options of a centralised or decentralised structure were discussed, looking at the advantages and disadvantages of both. The issue of mandatory versus compulsory staff development was considered, with the implications for the entire staff development process. Different implementation processes were outlined, using internal and external resources and identifying the characteristics of each. Finally, the issue of determining the financial accountability of staff development was discussed giving ways to justify expenditure.

REFERENCES

Dixon N Being intentional about organisation learning. In: Sofo F 1993 Strategies for developing a learning organisation. Training and Development in Australia September 25-28

Donovan J, Jackson A C 1991 Managing human service organisations. Prentice Hall, Sydney

Lee C 1988a Where does training belong. Training February: 53-60

Lee C 1988b Training budgets: neither boom nor bust. Training October: 41-46

Lowenthal W 1988 Continuing education for professionals: voluntary or mandatory. Journal of Higher Education 52:519-538

Pedler M, Burgoyne J, Boydell T 1991 The learning company. McGraw-Hill, London

Sofo F 1993 Strategies for developing a learning organisation. Training and Development in Australia September 25-28

6

Activities in staff development

Key questions

- What are the essential components of a position statement?
- How do you conduct an effective selection interview?
- What is a skills audit and how is it conducted?
- What is competency-based performance?
- How can you design a staff development program?
- How do you effectively manage an exit interview?

Content summary

Introduction

Recruitment—selection—appointment

Selection tools and techniques

Profiling techniques

Reaching a decision

Orientation-consolidation-continuing education

Needs assessment

Skills audit

Competency-based assessment
    Program design
    Program design and development
    Evaluation

Promotion-exit
    Feedback
    Promotion
    Exit
    References
    Career counselling

References

Introduction

Now you have an understanding of the staff development process and how to implement it into an organisation. The next step is to consider some key activities in the management and/or implementation of a staff development process. Your responsibilities may only be for some aspects of the process or for the entire process. In this chapter, activities are associated with particular stages of the process, but it should be recognised that activities and stages flow into one another and can occur individually or in combination. Where appropriate, examples will be given.

Recruitment–selection–appointment

Key activities within these stages are often considered part of the personnel functions of the organisation. An organisation may have a personnel department or relevant activities may be dealt with by a divisional manager. In a decentralised organisation, the activities will likely be dealt with by the manager of the department, unit or area.

Position statements (job description)

Every position in an organisation should have a position statement. Unfortunately, in some health care organisations today position statements do not necessarily exist, even though at some time some one must have identified the parameters of the position and the skills and abilities required for that position to create it.

A position statement is developed from a position analysis, so in terms of understanding what makes a good position statement it is useful to consider this analysis process.

Step 1: Define how the job should be done

- Develop a list of the key elements of the position.
- Identify the tasks that make up each element.
- Observe other employees in such positions noting how they do the job.
- Discuss the position with employees and find out from them what they do and what in their opinion is most significant and why.
- Ask other managers about the position and get them to identify the elements of the position.
- Study existing position statements and analyse their accuracy/relevance at this time.
- Identify the performance priorities of the position.

Step 2: Define the individual elements of the position

- Break each element down into specific tasks—how should things be done.
- Observe other employees, taking particular note of elements of the position.

- Discuss observations with employees.
- Challenge existing statements and opinions.
- Look for new ideas and improvements.

Step 3: Determine required standards for each element

- Review overall (organisation) standards in relation to this position.
- Determine how performance can be demonstrated.
- Clarify priorities, developing essential and preferred performance standards.
- Obtain feedback from employees and peers on the standards that have been determined.

Step 4: Write the position statement

- Write simply and clearly.
- Use headings and subheadings to organise content.
- Content should include the name of the position and nominate the reporting mechanism; state the function/purpose; state duties and responsibilities; identify areas (and people) of responsibility; identify relationships, working conditions, essential and preferred qualifications; identify how performance is to be measured.

Position statements have some limitations. They tend to be activity oriented rather than result oriented; that is, they detail what an employee does rather than the results to be achieved. Therefore, they should be viewed as a starting place in the development of performance expectations. Position statements sometimes limit performance in that an employee may avoid or refuse to do something because it is not in the position statement. To overcome this, the last item of the statement of responsibilities might read, *all other appropriate and reasonable duties that may be asked from time to time*. This provides some flexibility for the organisation.

Here is a sample (fictitious) position statement showing key headings/ structure:

Western Districts Health Service
Position statement

Title:	Education program manager
Division:	Clinical services
Location:	Shelley, Perth WA
Responsible to:	Manager clinical services
Salary:	Negotiable package
Date:	1 May 1995
Job purpose:	Lead the development, management and marketing of staff education throughout the organisation

---

Key outcomes areas

1 Provide education services which meet group needs.
2 Assess learning needs of all staff.
3 Evaluate options for intervention.
4 Develop strategies with particular emphasis on excellence
` in performance.
5 Conduct education and development programs.
6 Evaluate the effectiveness of interventions.
7 Establish outside markets for programs.

Job complexity

Setting priorities and managing time in a situation where there may be conflicting demands for services. Identifying the underlying needs and the most appropriate course of action given constraints of cost and time.

Job responsibilities

1 Conduct programs and deal with staff in a manner consistent with the professional ethics and organisational philosophy and policy.
2 Estimate costs of options to give line managers
   realistic assessment of their commitment.
3 Review and revise position responsibilities.
4 Conduct ongoing needs assessment.
5 Negotiate to determine priorities and recommend options
   for consideration by line managers.
6 Appraise participation against established standards.

Selection criteria

Essential knowledge and skills:
Registration as a nurse; a higher degree in nursing, education or a related discipline
Demonstrated competence in marketing strategies
Evidence of leadership ability
Demonstrated competence in education presentation, program design and development, administration and financial management
High level of interpersonal skills
Knowledge of health care issues
Commitment to the philosophy of the organisation
Additional desirable knowledge and skills:
Computer literacy
Experience in the development of self—directed education
Experience in adult education

Advertisements

We have all read advertisements that have presented a position as very interesting and attractive. For example:

> This senior position offers an outstanding opportunity to be at the leading edge of health care change within Australia. Based in Melbourne, you will be working with one of the country's leading teaching hospitals that is changing the paradigm of delivering health care. The hospital offers an excellent working environment and a genuine commitment to superior patient care and customer service (Weekend Australian 19 November, 1994).

An advertisement aims to attract applications, to catch the eye of the reader. In writing a good advertisement, it is useful to focus on what you think the reader will be looking for:

* some information or idea about the organisation
* a clear statement of the position
* the parameters of the role
* required qualifications and experience
* desirable qualifications and experience
* an indication of conditions including remuneration
* a contact for further information and application.

The organisation obviously wants people to be attracted to the advertisement and to apply but does not want to be swamped by inappropriate applications. Therefore, a good advertisement acts as a sifting agent. Many organisations now hire firms to recruit and select for positions. This means that the advertisement is usually restricted in its information about the organisation. Organisations justify this third party approach believing it is buying specialised expertise. The third party must take the responsibility for answering queries and giving out information as negotiated. Although I support the use of specialists for recruitment and selection, I am not convinced that keeping the organisation's name a secret until interview has merit. It is far more difficult to tailor an application appropriately to an unknown employer, and this approach can disadvantage the applicant.

I believe there is some essential information and some desirable information in a good advertisement. The essential information should include:

* the name of the position
* the name of the organisation (employer)
* a statement about the position
* a statement about accountability
* essential qualifications and experience
* desirable (preferred) qualifications and experience
* a statement of conditions (salary or salary negotiations, location)
* contact details.

Desirable information includes:

- information about the organisation (employer)
- time of the appointment (immediate start or whenever)
- assistance with relocation (if appropriate)
- information about the industry.

In terms of the structure of the advertisement, it should be informative but not verbose. Lists of points of information read better than long paragraphs and the essential information is clearer. An attractive advertisement might elicit the following reactions from the reader:

That looks really interesting. I have found the perfect job for me. I can do all that.

Now there is a challenging position. I'd love to give that a go. This has been written for me.

While these fictitious advertisements below meet most of the requirements of an effective advertisement neither is particularly exciting and the wording and terms (for example, wages) leave something to be desired.

Family Conflict Resolution Service, WA

FAMILY THERAPIST
(Sessional, Part-time or Full-time)

Salary range up to $40,000 (or pro rata)
Applications in writing are sought regarding the following position(s), sessional, part-time or full-time, becoming vacant in December 1993.
Contact: Mary Jones, Co-ordinator, Family Conflict Resolution Service on (09) 4574172 for further information and/or job description.
This agency is a service funded by the Federal Attorney General's Department as part of the Federal Government's commitment to deal with family conflict and thereby lessen the risk of youth homelessness. Clients are from families in conflict. This may be to the point where actual or possible youth homelessness is an issue.
Both parties, parents/care givers and the young person are engaged in the counselling process.
The position: Family therapy and mediation will be conducted under the supervision of the Co-ordinator under conditions approved and accredited by the Federal Attorney General's Department.
The person: Formal qualifications, experience and skills required in the areas of psychology or social work or other related professional areas eligible for registration in WA. Applicants should be willing to continue to develop their professional skills.
Applications to: The Director, Family Conflict Resolution Services, WA PO Box 999, Shelley WA 6148
Closing date: 5 PM Friday 9 May 1995.

Health Department
Eastern Suburbs Health Service

CLINICAL NURSE-THEATRE/GENERALIST LEVEL 2

We have a vacancy for a Clinical Nurse with Operating Theatre experience. The position involves theatre work 0.4 and 0.6 general clinical nursing. The successful applicant will be responsible for the management of the operating theatre suite in the district Health Centre which has 25 acute beds with a significant proportion of the clientele presenting for surgical procedures. Visiting Specialists perform general, ophthalmic, orthopaedic, gynaecological and E.N.T. surgery for the Health Service.
Wages: The wage range for the position is between -
$660.20-$724.60 per week.
Written applications addressing the selection criteria, current Curriculum Vitae and the names and addresses and telephone numbers of two professional referees should be lodged with -
A/Director of Nursing, Eastern Suburbs Health Service
PO Box 239, Shelley WA 6148.
Closing date: 5pm Friday 4 May 1995.

The third example is a much more exciting advertisement and uses the third party approach. There are less specific details but the organisation and the position are presented in such an interesting way that anyone interested could not help but make further inquiries:

Nursing Executive
Staff Development Centre

Senior role focusing on staff development
research and development

This position offers an outstanding opportunity to be at the leading edge of health care change within Australia. Based in Perth, you will be working with one of the country's leading teaching hospitals which is changing the paradigm for delivering health service. The hospital offers an excellent working environment and a genuine commitment to uperior patient care and customer service.

Opportunity to advance your career with a major hospital
at the forefront of change

Reporting to the Nursing Executive Director, the key functions of the role will include the establishment of an integrated staff development centre which will provide the framework to meet both nursing and non-nursing development needs through a committee structure and the appointment of unit based educators.

You will be involved in establishing integrated and collaborative models of education, practice and research in partnership with the tertiary sector, as well as promoting education/staff development programs to the international market. To be successful you will be a registered nurse with a relevant. Postgraduate qualification and demonstrated research and program evaluation experience. You will have sound analytical and education administration skills with a track record in facilitating the education of others. The ability to think creatively, combined with excellent negotiating and interpersonal skills will also be key ingredients to your success.

Previous employment with the tertiary sector would be an advantage.

Interested individuals should mail or fax a resume to the address below quoting Ref. No. M2900

Telephone enquires on (09) 4570000
Westland Consultants, 200 Moss Street, Shelley WA 6148

Selection tools and techniques

Choosing someone for a position involves predicting or forecasting whether a candidate will fulfil the requirements of the position. There is always a risk involved in that decision. Predicting performance can be assisted by a number of tools, such as:

- profiling the person to identify their work and interpersonal style, strengths and weaknesses and preferred work patterns
- reviewing evidence such as references, qualifications, work history, reports, examples of work
- assessing the individual face-to-face, as at interview
- testing the individual with case studies, scenarios, problem solving questions
- observing the individual at interview and, if possible, at work.

Many people identify considerable difficulty and discomfort with either conducting an interview, or being interviewed. Preparation and practice is the best way to decrease concern.

Being an interviewer

Through a process of review and inquiry, you should bring a list of applicants down to a short list of possible successful applicants who then will present at an interview. As the interviewer, you should feel that all the applicants at this stage have a reasonable chance of being successful. There is nothing to be gained, considering your time and the outcome for the applicant, by interviewing an individual who has not met the criteria. The interview should be used as an opportunity to collect information not already obtained, to evaluate the applicant on an interpersonal level and to give the applicant a chance to expand in areas where they feel they have particular knowledge and/or expertise. It is a time of information sharing as well as judgement. The following guidelines will assist:

1   Choose the selection panel carefully; three is a useful number.
2   Review thoroughly all evidence you have prior to the interview.
3   Prepare a set of questions to elicit the information you want across a broad range of areas.
4   Apply a score grid to the questions to rate answers and apply scores consistently for each question for each candidate; total scores at the end of each interview.
5   Allow sufficient time for interviews; 30 to 45 minutes is most appropriate.
6   Allow time between interviews to discuss and consider each applicant.
7   Attend to the physical environment to maximise conditions for all parties.
8   Make an effort to place the applicant at ease at the beginning to maximise the outcome.
9   Focus on objective judgement but do not disregard intuition and *gut feeling*.
10 Avoid making any definitive judgements until all applicants have been interviewed.

Being interviewed

There is nothing quite as nerve racking as an interview for a job. No matter how well prepared you are, you will always feel a little nervous, anxious and unsettled. Remember, if you get to the interview stage, you have impressed and you do have a good chance of success. The following guidelines will assist:

1   Remember, this is *your* interview so take control.
2   If you have the chance, get someone to run a mock interview with you so you can practice answering questions and dealing with your nerves.
3   Give yourself plenty of time to make the appointment; if you are feeling very nervous, get someone to drive you there to wait until you finish.
4   Pay attention to your physical needs; for example, dress well but be comfortable.
5   Prepare some questions that you think might be asked and practise the answers.
6   Identify any areas of your application that you want to emphasise.
7   Make sure you are comfortable; have a glass of water handy and ask for it if necessary.
8   Take your time to think through and answer a question.
9   If you do not understand a question ask for it to be repeated; if necessary ask for it to be stated in a different way.
10 If you feel unsure with the way you answer a question, don't be afraid to say you were not sure if that is what they were looking for with that question. If not, could they ask it again in a different way please.

11   If you feel really stumped by a question, admit it and ask for it to be restated differently and if necessary, admit you are not very sure of the answer.

12   Don't be afraid to ask your own questions.

13   You *always* have the right to ask about conditions, such as salary, holidays etc.

14   Remember, you will have done the best you could at the time. Don't evaluate yourself harshly afterwards, as there are rarely right and wrong answers to interview questions.

Profiling techniques

There are a number of programs available on the market offering a technique that *profiles* an individual. There are two parts to this technique. First, the organisation uses the tool to develop a *profile* of the (fictitious) best person for a position. Second, applicants are profiled and matched against the preferred profile. The *best match* should be the best candidate for the position. Typically, profiles comprise ratings of human traits such as interpersonal strengths, communication styles, decision making ability and style, work behaviour, preferred working style, personal characteristics and strengths. They are not the only tool however, and should be used as part of a package of tools. The act of developing the original profile can be the most useful part of the process in a situation where this has never been done before.

Reaching a decision

A decision can be made statistically, that is from the scores of each candidate. Or it can be judgemental; that is, from measurement plus personal judgement. Unquestionably, there is subjective judgement. We have all had experiences where we have had a feeling about a candidate which has influenced our decision. In most cases gut reaction should not be ignored, but recognised and considered. It is preferable however, that a judgement is supported by evidence. A good decision will be based upon *all* of the following:

- evidence (facts)
- experience
- potential
- presentation
- personal qualities
- the work place/position
- future projections
- intuition and feeling.

All applicants should be notified of the outcome of their interview and those who were unsuccessful should be offered an opportunity to discuss strengths and weaknesses. Feedback is crucial for the individual who has been unsuccessful. The successful applicant is usually notified verbally: *I am pleased to be able to offer you the position of....* or, *Congratulations, you are the successful applicant.*

The successful applicant is then notified in writing through a letter of appointment which should clearly identify the position and the conditions. This letter of appointment formally creates the relationship between employer and employee. It is preferable for the individual to reply formally in writing accepting the conditions of the position.

Orientation–consolidation–continuing education

The key staff development activities within these sections are traditionally viewed as staff development in that most activities relate to education/training. In terms of the process, the link between initial appointment and orientation-consolidation-continuing education is obvious, but the link between appointment to a new position, either as a promotion or career move, back to orientation-consolidation-continuing education is not as obvious. Again, an organisation may have allocated responsibility for these activities associated with these stages to a centralised department or responsibility may rest with individual departments. Regardless of the arrangement, the common activities within these three areas are discussed.

Needs assessment

Needs assessment has been discussed in detail within Chapter 2 and you may choose to review this before proceeding further. In terms of activities, it is useful to consider needs assessment in two ways: first, needs assessment for an individual and second, needs assessment for an organisation.

At the individual level, specific needs may have already been identified at initial interview and appointment. As part of the orientation process, it is useful to clarify needs as the individual may have had time to think more about the position or to identify further needs. For this purpose the following questions might be asked:

- Are there areas in the position where you feel your knowledge could be increased or improved?
- In what aspects of the job do you feel you could acquire more information?
- What would you like to know more about to enable you to improve your performance?
- What skills do you feel you could expand to enhance your performance?
- Are there any areas of this position when you feel unsure or lacking in experience?

Needs may be identified in a number of areas; for example, clinical practice, client condition, interpersonal skills, organisational structure and/or function, professional issues, specific elements of the job or work management.

Any of these questions could be relevant at any orientation; that is, for a new appointment or for a promotion or appointment to a new position.

At an organisational level, it may be decided to conduct a needs assessment within a department if there has been an expansion of service, or as part of continuing education initiatives. To facilitate the management of larger quantities of data, questions may be presented in a Likert scale such as the one below.

Job-related knowledge

In terms of your job, how important is it that you learn more about these topics at this time? For each statement below circle the number on the scale of 1-6 that best describes your view.

Very important	*VI*	*1*
Moderately important	*MI*	*2*
Important	*I*	*3*
Not important	*NI*	*4*
Moderately not important	*MNI*	*5*
Significantly not important	*SNI*	*6*

	VI	*MI*	*I*	*NI*	*MNI*	*SNI*
Personal time management	*1*	*2*	*3*	*4*	*5*	*6*
Negotiating skills	*1*	*2*	*3*	*4*	*5*	*6*
Current client conditions	*1*	*2*	*3*	*4*	*5*	*6*
Coping with dying and death	*1*	*2*	*3*	*4*	*5*	*6*
Performance evaluation	*1*	*2*	*3*	*4*	*5*	*6*
The ageing process	*1*	*2*	*3*	*4*	*5*	*6*
Pain management	*1*	*2*	*3*	*4*	*5*	*6*
Pharmacology	*1*	*2*	*3*	*4*	*5*	*6*

It may be necessary to provide an opportunity to elaborate on a particular area, for example, client conditions. This could be achieved in this way:

Client conditions

*If you marked a client condition as **MODERATELY OR VERY IMPORTANT** please provide further details. For example, **MULTIPLE SCLEROSIS**, list **FIVE** topics, for example, **symptoms, treatment**.*

Client condition is:

— —

List of topics

1 ....
2 ....
3 ....
4 ....
5 ....

Analysis of feedback can identify both broad and specific needs. It is advisable at this stage to feed your analysis back to respondents to have your results clarified and verified. This type of feedback, in which respondents can see what other people have identified can also prompt further discussion and expand information. As has been indicated earlier, needs assessment is not a one—off activity. It should be part of all performance reviews and an ongoing part of staff feedback.

Skills audit

Health care in Australia has undergone significant change in the past ten years and even more change in the future can be expected. Health care structures and organisations have been reviewed and restructured again and again in an effort to improve efficiency, cut costs, and respond to economic and/or political change. Sometimes changes occur in response to a new management team, the latest management model, or because of changes to staff expertise.

An organisation must remain aware of the skills in their workforce to be able to function effectively, recognising that the workforce is under constant change as individuals move in and out of positions. A skills audit is a means of identifying the skills currently held and the skills required by a workforce, so that an organisation can identify the complete range of skills at their disposal and identify any deficiencies. For example, a hospital may be planning to introduce a home care nursing service for surgical clients in response to early discharge policies that have resulted from the relocation of funding. Before commencing this service, the organisation needs to identify if they have nurses with sufficient experience and expertise (skills) to provide such independent nursing care when they will be more autonomous and have access to fewer resources. Another example is where an organisation decides to adopt a decentralised management model and to devolve responsibility for physical, financial and human resources. Before doing so, it would be wise to conduct a skills audit to establish if staff are able to function in this new role with this expanded level of accountability. Unfortunately, the importance of assessment before a decision is made is not always recognised nor included within planning.

A skills audit is a systematic process which identifies the present stock of skills or competencies held by the workforce, whether or not they are being actively used (i.e what is) and compares these with the skills or competencies that are needed (i.e what should be) (Clark 1990). The aims of a skills audit are similar to those of a financial audit or stocktake, in that it attempts to find out what is actually present and compares this with what ought to be present. Skills audits should exhibit the following features (Windsor 1991):

- a clear set of objectives that link skills to industry/enterprise/organisation strategy and changes
- quantifiable outcomes
- dates set for completion
- dates set for review.

Example: to provide more enriching and fulfilling jobs; to develop high job motivation in employees; to be conducted over three months starting from the first of next month.

- a well-defined, step-by-step process which is readily understood by all parties
- the use of more than one method of data collection to obtain full information, including questionnaire, interview, group process, observation and description.

Example: following consultation, a group process method to generate a list of skill requirements; followedup by a questionnaire to identify skills possessed.

- timely consultation with all parties from the beginning to end of the project, paying attention to different work patterns of staff, shifts, open discussion.

Example: morning, afternoon and evening groups to accommodate all staff.

- a procedure for reporting outcomes
- objective quantified data which identifies breadth and depth of responses, presented to all staff either in groups or through teams and/or managers.

Example: tables and graphs to show data analysis, presented to like groups of staff who are then given the opportunity to discuss and question the information.

- job re-design methods (if necessary)
- an open approach to the modification of existing positions to improve performance and increase quality of work life.

Example: data identifies that some staff in a particular area have skills that are not being utilised; positions are modified to allow for the utilisation of these skills.

- on going skills monitoring
- a tangible record is provided that may be useful both now and later but the process must be repeated.

Example: a skills audit is constructed within the same month each year to coincide with corporate planning.

Here is an example of a skills audit approach (Clark 1990):

Skills audit approach

- Preliminary meetings
- Group meetings   consultative
                                         steering committee
- Informal observation
- Development of data collecting instrument
- Data collection
- Analysis of data
- Reporting

The process may be conducted by people within the organisation or outside consultants may be utilised for some or all of the steps. The process must, however, be driven from within so that the stakeholders can own the outcomes. There are a number of possible outcomes of a skills audit:

- identification of strengths and weaknesses
- education for existing staff
- employment of new staff
- changes to roles and responsibilities
- modification of organisation plans
- maintenance of the status quo.

All outcomes will contribute to a better understanding of the workforce.

Competency-based assessment

During this phase of staff development, the focus tends to be more on performance and particularly on the assessment of performance to:

- advise the individual of their current level of performance and the individual's rate of progress towards the achievement of competency standards
- help the individual and others determine education needs
- determine if a unit of performance (competency) has been achieved for the purpose of formal recognition of expertise
- determine whether a person has achieved standards of performance (competency) which have not yet been recognised.

Competency-based assessment of performance is now the preferred method of establishing standards for and evaluating performance, and is particularly common in the health care sector. For this reason, there is considerable discussion on this topic. Competency standards have been developed, or are being developed, in most of the health professions. In nursing, for example, competency-based assessment determines eligibility for registration as well as a measure of advanced (expert) performance (ANCI 1993).

Competency comprises the specification of the knowledge and skill and the application of the knowledge and skill to the standard of performance required in employment. It includes all aspects of work performance, including:

- performance at an acceptable level of skill
- organising tasks
- responding and reacting appropriately when things go wrong
- defining a role in the scheme of things at work
- transfer of skills and knowledge to new situations.

The process of confirming that an individual has achieved competence is *assessment*. Standards of performance must be established for the assessor to be able to recognise competencies gained by individuals for employment or for credentials. *Assessor* is not, however, a title of a position, but the name given to the person acting in an *assessment role*. The *assessment process* should be encompassed within the normal work environment and the individual being assessed, as well as the assessor, needs to understand the process of assessment clearly.

Competency-based assessment is best achieved if the assessment procedure is planned, implemented, reviewed and recorded. Effective *planning* provides a guide to the approach to the assessment process; where it will take place, who should do it and over what time. It is important to clarify the reason for the assessment, to review current policies and procedures, and to explain the time frame in which it will occur. The factors that need to be considered are included in the performance criteria (Competency standards body: National Training Board, 1992) as shown below:

Planning Assessment

Elements	Performance criteria
Identify assessment context	Purpose of assessment is discussed and confirmed. Current endorsed competency standards, learning outcomes or performance measures are identified and discussed. Establishment policies are discussed.
Establish required evidence	Evidence is consistent with performance. Amount and type of evidence is sufficient to validate assessment decisions. Evidence required is discussed and confirmed.
Select and explain the assessment procedure	Appropriate assessment techniques are selected. Guidelines (rules) are discussed. Assessment procedures (and appeal mechanisms are discussed.
Organise assessment	Resources are organised consistent with assessment requirements, including costs. Appropriate people are advised. Assessment environment is prepared to facilitate a fair, valid and reliable assessment. Assessor's competence is confirmed. Assessment arrangements are confirmed with the individual being assessed.

Implementation of the process follows planning. It is important to have sufficient evidence on which to base a valid and reliable judgement of an individual's competence. This requires the collection and noting of evidence in some form. Performance criteria are designed to provide a clear and simple guide for people making assessment decisions; that is, to determine if the individual has achieved the standard as described by the performance criteria. Assessment is a joint process and it is fundamental that two-way com–munication is maintained throughout all the steps.

Assessment

Elements	*Performance criteria*
Gather evidence	Evidence is consistent with agreed standards. Evidence is valid, reliable, and consistent with agreed requirements and assessment techniques. Evidence is documented according to requirements.
Make the assessment decision	Assessment decision is based on evidence. Assessment decision is made in accordance with outcomes specified in competency standards, or performance measures and discussed and confirmed with the individual. Assessment decision is in accordance with the requirements of techniques.
Provide feedback during assessment	Establish comfort and ease. Progress is discussed during the process. Encouragement is given during the process.

The process of assessment is not complete until outcomes have been *recorded* and communicated to the parties involved in the assessment. It is a dynamic process and should be subject to constant review. As with assessment itself, the review should be a joint activity. With the growth of competency-based training many people will participate in the assessment processes on a regular basis. Evaluation and review of all aspects of the process is an essential requirement.

Recording assessment results

Elements	Performance criteria
Record assessment results	Results are recorded in co-operation with the person who has been assessed and in accordance with policies/requirements. Records as formal documents are stored appropriately.
Provide feedback to person being assessed	Performance is discussed and confirmed. Clear and constructive feedback is given. Person being assessed is encouraged to explore ways of overcoming gaps in competence. Person being assessed is advised of development opportunities.
Procedure is reviewed	Assessment procedure is reviewed by individuals involved and other relevant persons. Changes are made to procedures in light of review.

There are various **methods** of determining achievement, that is, of making an assessment. Assessment methods must be appropriate to the situation, the conditions, and the expected performance to be assessed. There are a number of different methods:

- observation of the individual completing a particular skill which may be accompanied by questions
- a structured practical demonstration with return performance; the observer (third party) sees the process and the outcome
- written testing to measure knowledge; may be used to complement a practical demonstration
- oral testing as an adjunct to practical demonstration or to test speed and accuracy of recall; useful when these are an essential component of competence
- projects completed without interference, when the outcome is used as the evidence
- simulations including computer simulations and role play where the event is similar to real life situations
- personal portfolios with examples of work, which can be useful to assess achievements

- computer-based situations, taking the form of either question and answer and/or interaction.

An example of an assessor's checklist (Competency standards body: National Training Board, 1992) is provided here to illustrate how the stages discussed earlier can be incorporated into a useful form.

Competency-based assessment

Assessor's checklist
Step 1 Planning the assessment
What is the purpose of this assessment?
Performance criteria discussed with: *Date:*
Assessment policy discussed with: *Date:*

Step 2: Evidence required
What does the person have to do?
What does the person have to know?
Discussed and confirmed with: *Date:*

Step 3: How is the assessment to be done?
Discussed and confirmed with:Date:

Step 4: Checking
Materials   *Time(s) set*
Equipment   *Time(s) set*
People   *Time(s) set*
Place   *Time(s) set*

Carrying out the assessment
Performance   *OK*   *NOT OK*   *Date*   *Initials*
1
2
3

Record results
Date:
Informed and discussed   *Date*
Signed
Signed

Evaluation of process

There a four key principles of assessment. Assessment must be valid, reliable, fair and flexible. Each should be understood and applied within the assessment.

Validity

Competency assessments are valid when they assess what they claim to assess. Validity of assessment is achieved when assessors are fully aware of what is to be assessed, as indicated by the units of competency, learning outcomes and clearly defined performance criteria. Evidence is collected from activities and tasks that can be clearly related to the unit of competency or learning outcomes specified for the situation. There should also be sufficient evidence to demonstrate that the performance criteria have been met. The principles of validity are:

- Assessments should cover the range of skills and knowledge needed to demonstrate competence.
- Assessment of competence should be a process which integrates knowledge and skills with their practical application.
- Judgements to determine the individual's competence should, wherever practicable, be made on evidence gathered on a number of occasions and in a variety of contexts and situations.

Reliability

Reliable assessment uses methods and procedures which engender confidence that competency standards and their levels are interpreted and applied consistently from individual to individual and context to context. Without reliable assessments there can be no comparability of credentials. High quality competency standards are fundamental to reliability. The principles of reliability are:

- Assessment practices should be monitored and reviewed to ensure that there is consistency in the interpretation of evidence.
- Assessors must be competent in terms of the accepted standards (national/ governing body/professional group).

Flexibility

The assessment practices endorsed for the implementation of competency-based education should be flexible if they are to be appropriate for a range of delivery methods and sites, and needs of individuals. There is not necessarily a single approach or set of approaches to the assessment of competence. The principles of flexibility are:

- Assessment should cover both the on and off-the-job components of the situation.
- Assessment procedures should provide for the recognition of competence, not how, where or when it was acquired.
- Assessment procedures should be made accessible to individuals so that they can proceed readily from one competency standard to another.

Fairness

Assessment is fair if it does not disadvantage particular individuals. If individuals understand what is expected of them and what form assessment will take, and if assessment places all individuals on equal terms and supports their learning, it is fair. The principles of fairness are:

- Assessment practices and methods should be equitable to all groups of individuals.
- Assessment procedures and the criteria for judging performance should be made clear to all individuals seeking assessment.
- There should be a participative approach to the development of competency standards, where the standards are developed and agreed to over time.
- Opportunities should be provided to allow individuals to challenge assessments and provision should be available for reassessment.

In summary, competency-based assessment is gaining favour in all workplaces, in line with the National Training Agenda and developments within professions. It is now recognised as an effective measure of performance and is an integral part of staff development.

Program design

The effectiveness of a staff development process depends on the existence of a carefully planned overall program that pays attention to all stages of the process. The design of such a program can be approached in a number of ways. There is no best design as a program should be designed for the individual organisation and will depend upon such things as:

- staff categories, levels and numbers
- organisational structure and function
- management processes and models
- accountability structures and processes
- performance management systems
- context
- client characteristics.

Any staff development program must be part of a total organisation strategic plan and must be viewed as part of organisational behaviour and processes. Any program designed in isolation without due regard to all other factors is likely to be short lived and of questionable value. The following general questions are a useful way to begin to design a program:

- Where is the authority for the program; that is, how important is it to the organisation and where and how is the support demonstrated?
- What led to the development of this program; that is, on what need, evidence or research is it based?
- What is the program trying to achieve?
- What are the agreed objectives?

- What are the expected outcomes?
- What evidence exists to demonstrate that a program will produce the required results?
- Who is the target population and how clearly is this defined?
- What other factors, conditions, structures, and/or processes are relevant to this program?
- What other, if any, like programs have been implemented, and what were the results of such programs?
- Is there resistance to this program and if so, from whom and how will it be managed?

The answers to these questions will ensure that consideration has been given to all relevant matters before the details of the program are considered. Now consider some of the more specific questions that are relevant to the actual structure and content of the program.

Scope: who is the program for?

Is the program for all staff, specific categories of staff, specific departments, for implementation at specific stages of employment?

Structure: how will it be structured?

Will it be managed centrally, by division or department; will it be mandatory or needs based; will it be run internally or externally?

Staff: who will be implementing this program?

Will it be designated staff development staff, managers/supervisors, external consultants, peers or colleagues?

Standards: how will it be evaluated and against what criteria?

What outcomes are expected and desired?

Subject: what is the content?

What knowledge and skills will be taught and what methods will be used?

Two figures are presented here to demonstrate two different approaches.

The first model demonstrates a performance management approach and encompasses all stages of a staff development process (Fig. 6.1). Each stage could be developed to meet specific needs and/or groups of staff and each stage has the potential to be developed into specific content areas (Schneider 1986). This model starts with the establishment of standards and measures. At this time the purpose of the program is established in terms of the overall organisation. Second, expectations of performance are set and agreed to. The third stage is the establishment of a plan for the program where the details are addressed—who will lead (co-ordinate), make the decisions and organise, and

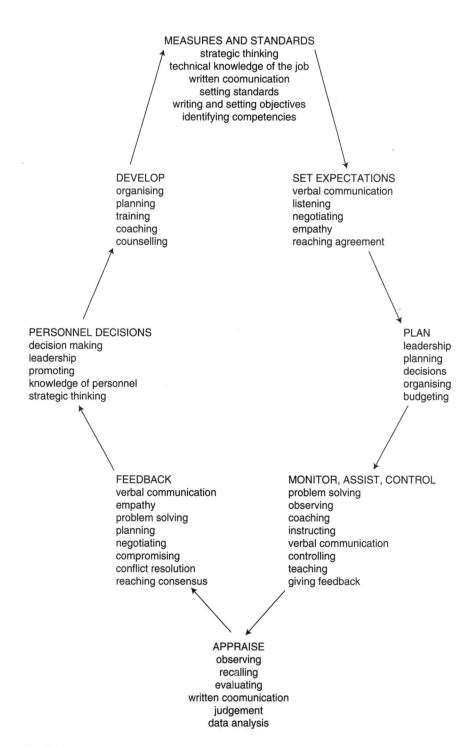

MEASURES AND STANDARDS
strategic thinking
technical knowledge of the job
written coomunication
setting standards
writing and setting objectives
identifying competencies

DEVELOP
organising
planning
training
coaching
counselling

SET EXPECTATIONS
verbal communication
listening
negotiating
empathy
reaching agreement

PERSONNEL DECISIONS
decision making
leadership
promoting
knowledge of personnel
strategic thinking

PLAN
leadership
planning
decisions
organising
budgeting

FEEDBACK
verbal communication
empathy
problem solving
planning
negotiating
compromising
conflict resolution
reaching consensus

MONITOR, ASSIST, CONTROL
problem solving
observing
coaching
instructing
verbal communication
controlling
teaching
giving feedback

APPRAISE
observing
recalling
evaluating
written coomunication
judgement
data analysis

Fig. 6.1 Performance management system

what are the budget constraints. The fourth stage involves the implementation of the program itself followed by the fifth stage, the appraisal of the program, through appraisal of performance. This information leads to stage six, the provision of feedback which may have an impact on a position (personnel) or the entire program, that is, stage seven. From these decisions further developments in the program may result, that is, stage eight, which will determine the relationship of the information to the established standards. So the cycle repeats itself. This model clearly links all the stages together and demonstrates the importance of thorough strategic planning. It is a good overall model for an organisation, without giving details of specific aspects of a program.

The second figure is an example of a program designed as part of an overall staff development program in a community based health care organisation (Fig. 6.2). This figure focuses on the orientation-consolidation-continuing education phase of the figure. It was developed for one category of staff, here called Care Aide, otherwise known throughout the health care system as personal carer, health worker, or personal care assistant. It was a workplace training scheme to be implemented throughout the entire organisation and was designed in accordance with the following principles:

- The training program was designed to meet the needs of the client population, organisation and the staff.
- The program recognised the characteristics of the employees so that adult learning principles were applied and recognition for prior learning and skill was given.
- The program was designed from the findings of a comprehensive needs assessment.
- Flexibility within activities was encouraged to meet individual needs.
- The training was competency-based to include emphasis on achievement of performance expectations, self directed activities, flexibility and recognition of ability.
- The program was based on a model of facilitated learning.
- The program was designed into modules of content, some of which were designated core modules and some optional modules, with some allowance for choice.
- Learning was sequential and built on expertise.

The program begins upon entry: that is, either at the beginning of year one (bottom of the figure), or at the beginning or year three.

- Two entry points for employees:
    Entry 1 = previously untrained
    Entry 2 = possesses a recognised qualification

- Three levels representing three years of employment:
    Level 1 = beginning performance (previously untrained)
    Level 2 = experienced performance
    Level 3 = advanced performance (possesses recognised qualification)

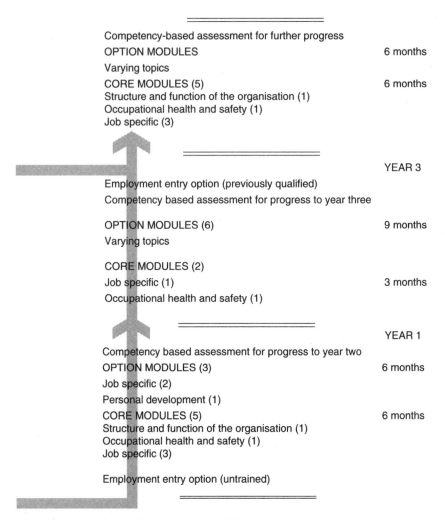

Competency-based assessment for further progress
OPTION MODULES   6 months
Varying topics
CORE MODULES (5)   6 months
Structure and function of the organisation (1)
Occupational health and safety (1)
Job specific (3)

                                                                 YEAR 3
Employment entry option (previously qualified)
Competency based assessment for progress to year three

OPTION MODULES (6)   9 months
Varying topics

CORE MODULES (2)
Job specific (1)   3 months
Occupational health and safety (1)

                                                                 YEAR 1
Competency based assessment for progress to year two
OPTION MODULES (3)   6 months
Job specific (2)
Personal development (1)
CORE MODULES (5)   6 months
Structure and function of the organisation (1)
Occupational health and safety (1)
Job specific (3)

Employment entry option (untrained)

Fig. 6.2 Community health worker (care aide) program

- Program is organised into modules. A module is a defined body of knowledge with clearly defined objectives and measurable outcomes.
- Modules vary in structure and may be on-the-job training; off-the-job training; self directed learning package; interactive video; computer assisted learning package; attendance at an approved course at a recognised institution.
- Modules are either:
  compulsory; for example, occupational health and safety, customer focus, organisation structure and function, job specific knowledge and/or skills
  optional; specific content, personal development, or be recommended by the employer.

Either model can be adapted for a particular organisation or employment category, but both represent an alternative approach to program design. There is no best model for a staff development program. The choice of model will be determined only after careful consideration of all the relevant factors. The following approach provides a useful guide:

Program design and development

1 Determine the parameters of the program:
   * organisation-wide (hospital)
   * department (nursing services)
   * employment classification (registered and enrolled nurses)
   * position (clinical nurse specialist).
2 Establish a clear purpose, overall and specific objectives and desired outcomes.
3 Consider all constraints, such as time, cost, expertise, resources and priorities.
4 Identify any possible problems and anticipate the effect they may have on the program:
   * unrealistic expectations of outcomes
   * management attitudes or restraints
   * previous experiences
   * staff attitudes.
5 Identify key personnel to be involved in discussion and development.
6 Develop an interim plan giving consideration to all relevant factors, including cost and obtain feedback from as many areas as possible.
7 Review, modify, amend as necessary.
8 Communicate the plan to relevant personnel well in advance to allow for planning.
9 Implement the program.
10 Evaluate.

Evaluation

Evaluation is a key component of any staff development program. Evaluation can be described as a process of description and judgement usually conducted to determine the effectiveness of a program. Effective evaluation depends on a clear statement of the objectives of the program which are then evaluated in the context of the specific activities of the program and in terms of the way the objectives are expressed.

Evaluation has a number of purposes many of which are interrelated:

* To identify problems within the program and locate the cause
* To ensure the program is relevant to stated objectives
* To test new approaches and identify their effect
* To provide justification for decisions or actions
* To provide feedback to individuals and the organisation.

Comprehensive evaluation will occur on a number of levels:

The philosophy or purpose of the organisation

Is the philosophy or purpose of the organisation clearly represented?

The objectives

Do the objectives specify the competencies expected of the employee; are the objectives being attained?

Administration and organisation

Who relates/reports to whom; how are relationships established and maintained; is the budget realistic; are the resources adequate?

Staffing (implementing the program)

Are the staff involved and appropriately qualified; are the staff committed?

Staff (recipients of the program)

Do staff achieve the expected outcomes; do staff indicate satisfaction; are individual needs addressed?

Content

Is the content relevant and appropriate for the organisation at this time; does the content require modification and/or change; are areas of knowledge and skill and personal development being addressed?

Resources, facilities, services

Are these appropriate, available, adequate?

No discussion on evaluation would be complete without reference to formative and summative evaluation as each provides different information. Formative evaluation provides information to make decisions about mod–ifications or developments in areas, process and materials. It best serves the developers, providers and decision makers, that is, those specifically involved in the implementation of the program. Summative evaluation, however, provides information for accepting or rejecting a program. It best reflects overall accountability.

In summary, evaluation is an integral component of any staff development program as it is of any staff development process. Evaluation can be conducted at a specific time, for a specific purpose, using specific instruments and can produce specific data. It can also be conducted as part of every process or activity that occurs. No results of an overall evaluation should be a surprise if a process of ongoing evaluation has been implemented.

Promotion–exit

The last group of key activities to be discussed occur most frequently during the promotion–exit phase of the staff development process. Promotion or exit can occur at any time of employment; therefore, it is the activities that occur in relation to the event rather than the event itself that are important.

A key activity throughout the entire staff development process involves the review of performance and this has been discussed in Chapter 4. Performance review involves the giving and receiving of feedback. These activities are fundamental to the effective review of performance.

Feedback

The ability to give and receive feedback depends on the nature of the relationship between the parties concerned. The importance of establishing a relationship between employer and employee has been identified as a key component of the staff development process. The relationship is important in a general sense but particularly important when it comes to evaluating performance.

Feedback is information provided to a person for the purpose of maintaining or improving performance (Hayes 1984). It is not advice, which is telling someone what they should do. The statement, *If I were you I would have done...* is probably one of the least useful statements ever made. You are not the other person and if you were, you would probably have done exactly what they did. Feedback is letting others know how their performance affects you and/or your area of responsibility. Successful feedback depends upon:

- the other person understanding the information
- the other person accepting the information
- the other person being able to do something with the information.

There are four types of feedback, neutral, positive, negative and nil feedback.

Neutral feedback

This is information with no expressed or implied quality dimension; it carries no judgement and provides no results. Assumptions are made that if performance is below expectation the employee will know, and that the employee will know how to bring performance into line; that circumstances leading to poor performance are within the control of the individual. Examples of neutral feedback include the numbers and types of client complaints, numbers and types of medication errors, and descriptive statements about poor staff performance within your department.

Positive feedback

This is information that has a positive quality factor built in, in the form of praise, salary increase, promotion, increased responsibility or autonomy, or special privileges. Recognition and praise of good performance encourages the performance and helps to create a positive environment. Examples of positive feedback include the numbers and types of client complaints, with acknowledgment of improvements and efforts of staff to learn from errors; number and types of medication errors as compared to last figures with recognition of education initiatives to improve the situation; statements that recognise improvements in staff performance and growth in team spirit and commitment, which is attributed to your management.

Negative feedback

This information is given with a built in negative quality factor. Corrective advice is given and a change in performance is required. Statements focus on identifying what is current, and on planning for a change in the future. Examples include, numbers and types of client complaints noting an increase in incidence and no attempt at improvement; statements about poor performance of staff within your area of responsibility and no apparent attempt on your part to make changes.

Nil feedback

No information is given, neither positive, negative nor neutral. Individuals have no way of measuring or evaluating performance. Apathy and lack of interest are common. The phrase, *no news is good news,* is not appropriate in terms of the review of performance. Staff should be advised of their performance and where they stand in relation to standards, expectations and past assessment.

Providing feedback

All levels of staff should give and receive feedback regardless of structures, management style or accountability. In any organisation with an open, honest change-oriented environment, staff will seek out feedback rather than wait to receive it. Feedback like appraisal should be informal and formal, continuous as well as specifically related to stages of employment.

General guidelines for providing feedback
- *Be selective:* reserve it for key issues or situations rather than nitpicking.
- *Be specific:* give precise information so the reason for feedback is clearly understood; avoid the terms always and never as they are generalisations and of little use.
- *Be prompt:* minimise the time lag between behaviour and feedback.
- *Be descriptive:* talk about what you see and hear and the impact on behaviour; focus on facts not conclusions.
- *Be sensitive:* be aware of the whole situation, work demands, the setting; even excellent feedback can be given at the wrong time and be harmful.
- *Be creative*: be prepared to broaden your vision and look for alternatives.

Guidelines for providing positive feedback

- *Be aware of your attitude:* avoid taking good performance for granted; recognise the needs of others and not just your own.
- *Be honest:* exaggeration of the significance of behaviour will embarrass; minimising achievement is insensitive.
- *Be open:* positive feedback should stand alone, not precede negative feedback; don't set people up.
- *Be clear:* qualifiers can ruin the effect of praise and may come across as condescending, downgrading and/or demeaning.

Guidelines for providing negative feedback

- *Be direct:* get to the point quickly using straight forward statements.
- *Be reactive:* seek out a reaction; make a statement and ask for a response; be prepared for defensiveness, blaming or refusal to accept; be empathic and understanding but avoid the need to argue and justify; depend on your evidence
- *Be consultative:* aim for at least a partial agreement, but demand compliance with acceptable standards if agreement can not be reached.

After negative feedback has been given and reacted to, set about developing a plan to achieve small steps towards resolution, accepting slow progress. Summarise by restating to confirm understanding. Finally, follow up and set a date for review and make sure you keep it.

Guidelines for receiving feedback

Receiving feedback can make a substantial contribution to your growth and development. Look for opportunities to elicit feedback from superiors, peers, colleagues and clients.

- *Don't hang the messenger:* avoid a reaction that can be interpreted as retaliation, remain open and fight defensiveness.
- *Understand what you have been told:* ask questions, request examples, affirm meaning.
- *Check the information:* increase your insight by seeking out responses from others.
- *Determine what to do with the information*: implement action based on information.

You have a right to choose your behaviour and a responsibility to accept the consequences. Select the areas that make most sense to you and that you wish to work on then plan changes to behaviour and look for evidence to confirm growth. Some individuals spend considerable energy trying to change their behaviour for someone else, when the required behaviour is just not possible. If you cannot change, accept the consequences of your decision and avoid unnecessary failure.

The key to feedback is the simple notion of respect for the employee as a person. Feedback is not an excuse for demeaning and embarrassing someone in front of others. Most people want to be effective and feedback is an important component of effectiveness. *If I have done well reward me. If I have done badly, then tell me—but let me know I have the capacity to make it the next time* (Hunt 1986).

Promotion

Promotional positions are not always available but opportunities should be made available wherever possible. Potential for promotion is often recognised within the context of staff education and development and it is often the person in staff development who recognises the potential of an individual. Promotion is usually viewed as a reward—an acknowledgment of performance. It may include the recognition of potential, an opportunity for expansion of expertise, or a requirement of the organisation to meet a change in structure or function or service.

It is essential to recognise that any move to a new position, promotional or otherwise, requires a return to the orientation-consolidation-continuing education phase of staff development. Promotion to a more senior position should not be seen as an independent event and must be viewed within the context of the entire process.

Promotion usually brings about intrinsic and extrinsic rewards. Intrinsic rewards include challenge, power, recognition, autonomy and/or creativity. Extrinsic rewards include salary increase, bonuses, insurance, fringe benefits, or an increase or change in resources. Promotion may mean different things to different people and assumptions should not be made about the value of a promotion. As a reward, it will be most effective if the individual is able to satisfy their intrinsic and extrinsic needs. When consideration is being given to a promotion, all the activities associated with recruitment-selection-appointment are relevant. Activities may be handled internally but they are no less important than in any other position.

Exit

Because of the relationship that often develops between staff in general and staff with staff development responsibilities, it is often the staff development person who is first told of an individual's intention to leave an organisation. Staff may leave a place of employment for a number of reasons: as a career choice, retirement by choice, termination by employer direction, or retrenchment. Regardless of the reason for the departure, exit from employment, at particular organisation brings about a series of staff related activities. The key activities to be discussed are provision of exit interviews, references and career counselling. First, it is useful to further discuss the four reasons for exit as outlined above.

Career choice

Some individuals will choose to stay in the same position with the same employer for most if not all their working life. They grow and change with the position and over time, becoming part of the organisation. Other individuals will stay for relatively short periods, preferring to pursue new challenges, or experience changes in career directions. Some individuals move on in response to family, partner, economic or personal situations and some just never settle anywhere. All individuals contribute to an organisation and no opportunity should be lost to learn from an employee's experiences and ideas and to obtain constructive criticism. The individual who leaves an organisation by choice takes considerable knowledge and skill with them, obtained during their employment. They may have cost the organisation in terms of education and other resources and the organisation would usually rather not lose the individual and the investment. But if an individual chooses to leave, there is little to be gained from making the exit difficult. Both employee and employer need to bring the employment contract to a conclusion.

Voluntary retirement

Smart individuals plan retirement, adjusting their life style over time to facilitate a smooth transition. Many people report being busier after retirement than they were when they worked and retirement certainly does not mean the end of stimulating activities. However, few individuals will retire from employment without feelings of apprehension, anxiety, excitement and/or relief. Again, someone retiring from an organisation can be a source of very useful information and may feel particularly able to be very honest in their comments. Again, both employee and employer need to bring the employment contract to a conclusion.

Termination

Termination of employment as a result of poor performance or disciplinary action is never pleasant. Hopefully, the process that has resulted in this action has included appraisal, feedback, counsel and an appropriate system of advice (warning). Comprehensive documentation is essential. In this case the employee and employer have certain rights and timely access to internal and external resources and services can prove to be very useful. Regardless of the nature of the situation, if handled well, there is still room for growth and learning for all concerned.

Retrenchment

What ever term you use—downsizing, retrenchment, letting people go—the reality of large or small scale sacking is uncomfortable for everyone. There is the issue of the unpleasant task of sacking the staff, and also dealing with the morale of the staff who remain. There have been horror stories of mass sackings in some industries in recent years but the health industry has not had the same numbers involved. Stories of memos that read, *Dear staff member, Your services are/are not required as of today...*, with a line through one of the options, indicate a complete disregard for the most basic employee rights of courtesy, respect and consideration. Organisations may use an outplacement agency and offer career and personal counselling, career planning and stress management strategies. They advise individuals of their entitlements, the opportunities that exist, and provide advice on application and interview for other positions. Retrenchment can never be pleasant, but it can be managed well with minimum negative effect and even can facilitate a positive career move.

Exit interview

All of the points discussed in the sections on being interviewed and being an interviewer have relevance here. The atmosphere, physical environment, structures and process are all important. There are some specific points that warrant discussion.

- Establish the purpose clearly as far in advance as possible to allow for preparation and to set the expectations. For example, *This interview offers an opportunity for you to comment on any aspect of the organisation or your position. Your constructive criticism is very welcome.*
- Prepare some general questions and some specific questions if you have specific needs. For example, What do you think are the strengths and weaknesses of this organisation? How could your position be better structured to produce best performance?
- Allow plenty of opportunity for the individual to talk, and listen well. For example, *What would you like to tell me?*
- Avoid conflict and try not to respond to emotional outbursts or accusations. For example, *I appreciate this is a difficult time for you, but I believe we can both learn if we remain calm.*
- Ask about future plans and be prepared to refer to resources that may be available. For example, *What plans do you have for the future? Have you discussed these with the following?*
- Acknowledge performance and achievement and where appropriate, indicate their contribution to the organisation. For example, *You have been a valued member of the staff and your contribution to the organisation is appreciated.*

The following guidelines may help to minimise the inevitable unpleasantness of having to terminate someone's employment. It is most likely that someone in a senior management position will have the responsibility but you may be required to also be involved:

- Have two people present at the interview, as well as the employee.
- Review all documentation and processes that have occurred and be sure of the facts of the matter and that appropriate policies have been adhered to.
- Prepare what you are going to say and have a statement in writing with a letter of advice.
- Be prepared for an emotional outburst which could be anger, denial, non acceptance or distress.
- Avoid a lengthy debate or discussion and refrain from justifying and defending your decision, beyond a fair explanation.
- Plan the announcement of your decision to appropriate staff and advise those directly affected by your decision.

References

References can be completely useless or can contribute significantly to the data collected on an applicant. It is unlikely that anyone would ask a person to be a referee, if they were not sure of a positive result. Therefore, references are sometimes considered to be of little value. If the application asks for the name and contact details of a referees, you should seek a reference. It is not unusual to obtain a reference over the telephone and to record it as a verbal reference. For your benefit and for theirs, have questions prepared and seek the information you need to know. Questions may be general and be asked for all applicants, or may be specific to elicit information about a specific individual. Ask for examples of behaviour or abilities and gather specific details where possible. Allow for open discussion, for example, *Is there anything in particular you would like to comment on?*

If, on the other hand, you are asked to provide a written reference, the following guidelines may be useful:

- Obtain information about the position, for example, the position statement.
- Make reference to the responsibilities of the position.
- Emphasise strengths and minimise any shortcomings.
- Be honest, you do no one a favour by gilding the lily, least of all, the applicant.
- Try to be objective but do not ignore your personal judgement.
- Where possible, give examples.
- Be prepared to comment further if required.

If you feel uncomfortable about being a referee, decline rather than struggle to be objective.

Career counselling

Career counselling is, in the main, facilitated goal setting. It is often difficult to examine your options realistically and to consider your strengths and short comings objectively. Someone who can ask the right questions, challenge you to examine your goals and aspirations, and comment honestly on your abilities is of great value. Frequently the counsellor has no answers but assists the individual to come to the best decision at the time. There are many factors, economic, social, personal and/or professional, that will affect your decision. The focus of career counselling discussions should be to:

- analyse the current situation
- identify all the relevant factors involved
- identify short and long term goals
- recognise all the options
- establish realistic strategies
- identify resources present and needed
- make a decision (or agree to not make a decision at this time)
- resolve unfinished business.

In summary, a promotion in or exit from employment can be a significant turning point in an individual's working life. It can also be a useful time for employer and employee and even the most difficult time can be resolved productively.

Chapter summary

This chapter has taken a comprehensive look at many different activities that occur within the staff development process. Activities have been discussed within the sections of the process where they are most likely to occur, but individual activities may occur throughout the process. In the recruitment-selection-appointment stage of the process, the focus was on obtaining the best person for the job. In the orientation-consolidation-continuing education state of the process, the focus was on collecting data, assessing performance, developing a program from identified needs, and evaluating the outcomes of a program. In the promotion-exit stage of the process the focus was on the relationship between employer and employee, the giving and receiving of feedback, and obtaining useful information from staff during employment, and particularly when they leave.

REFERENCES

ANCI 1993 Australian Nursing Council: National competencies for the registered and enrolled nurse in recommended domains. ANC

Clark T W 1990 Getting to grips with skills audits. TAFE National Centre for Research and Development, South Australia

Competency standards body 1992 Workplace trainers. National Training Board, Canberra

Hayes M 1984 Managing performance: a comprehensive guide to effective supervision. Lifetime Learning Publications Belmont, California

Hunt J W 1986 Managing people at work. McGraw-Hill Book Company, London

Schneider C 1986 Creating a performance management system. Training and Development Journal, May 74-79

Windsor K 1991 Skills counts: how to conduct gender-bias free skills audits. Australian Government Publishing Service, Canberra

7

Methods to achieve staff development outcomes

Key questions

- How do you choose the right method?
- How do you plan a staff development presentation?
- How can you effectively deliver an interactive presentation?
- What are the advantages of self-directed methods?
- What is the real value to an organisation of a conference or convention?
- What place do train-the-trainer programs have in staff development?
- How do you deliver a meaningful presentation?

Content summary

Introduction

There are as many different ways to achieve staff development outcomes as there are different topics and the choice of any one method will depend upon a number of factors. The principles behind the best choice for a situation should be to obtain the maximum result, to have the greatest impact, or to bring about a behaviour change that is a result of growth and development. This chapter will discuss different methods using specific examples.

Choosing a method

How do you determine what is the best method for a situation? Good decisions will be made if the situation is appraised from a number of perspectives. First, examine the context of the situation, considering such factors as:

- what you are aiming to achieve
- why is action necessary/needed
- who is involved
- how does the situation fit into the overall plan
- what are the resource implications
- what is the time frame.

Second, examine the participants considering such factors as:

- the needs of the individuals
- how many are involved
- whether it is a homogeneous group
- whether staff are at the same level and/or classification
- how staff have become involved
- their backgrounds
- what the individuals want to achieve
- how outcomes will be measured.

Third, examine the topic or subject, considering such things as:

- what they believe they need to know
- what you believe they need to know
- the parameters of the topic/subject
- whether this is a once-only session or part of a series, or part of a larger topic
- whether the topic lends itself to a particular method

The following examples will demonstrate how different methods can be implemented effectively.

Example 1: Developing skills for interviewing and selecting staff

A group of middle level managers have been designated responsibility for interviewing and selecting staff in their department. This responsibility is part of a recently acquired personnel responsibility in line with the organisation's management restructuring. There have been no additional resources allocated to facilitate this development and it is a matter of some urgency as the practice will begin as soon as necessary; that is, when staff are needed. There are eight managers in the group affected by this decision and skill and experience varies considerably. They all know they need some development in the area and that appraisal of their performance will consider this aspect of their role. The group needs to develop skills in writing job descriptions (statements), writing advertisements, developing selection criteria, reviewing applications, conducting interviews, analysis and decision making, and giving feedback. You decide that a four step approach will be most effective.

Developing skills for interviewing and selecting staff

Step 1 Hold a 2-hour session with some teaching and some discussion.
         Distribute pre-reading material.
         Distribute exercises to take away and work on.

Step 2 Hold a 3-hour session to discuss exercises and give feedback.
         Encourage role playing of situations.

Step 3 Individualise follow-up by you as a mentor when a manager has
         to put new learning into effect.

Step 4 Plan a 1-hour session for when individuals will have had some
         experience and can discuss situations and obtain feedback from
         each other.

Example 2: Developing clinical skills

There has been a change in a clinical procedure on a ward. Some staff have experience but quite a few do not. It is a relatively common procedure so learning needs to occur as soon as possible. There is plenty of opportunity for learning during normal work time and there are sufficient resources available to implement clinical teaching. You consult with the designated manager and propose a four step approach.

Developing clinical skills

Step 1 Identify staff with experience and those who need to learn the
         procedure.
         Establish that a common protocol exists which is documented
         and has been accepted by appropriate personnel.
         Establish required levels of competence and methods
         of assessment.

Step 2 Facilitate a clinical learning session with the experienced staff
         so they can work through the procedure and establish common
         understanding and practice.
         Ensure a commitment to take on a preceptor role by the
         experienced staff.
         Work through the preceptor role with them.

Step 3   *Match up (buddy) experienced and inexperienced staff and ask them to work out how they will conduct their clinical learning session*

              Follow-up to ensure planning has occurred; be prepared to deal with the situation if buddies can not work together

Part 4   *Establish a mechanism for review and arrange for evaluation and feedback from participants.*

Example 3: An opportunity for staff to attend an international conference on the management of health services in Australia in the future

Within the organisation's staff development budget there are sufficient funds to send three staff to a 3-day conference in a (another) capital city in Australia. There are a number of staff who have either indicated an interest or who would, you believe, benefit from this conference. You determine which staff are the most appropriate delegates considering their current position and responsibility within the organisation. You clarify for yourself the content of the program, the quality/experience of the presenters and the format. Following discussion with other staff at a management meeting, you determine this approach:

Selecting staff for attendance at a national conference

Step 1   *Develop criteria for attendance; for example: has not attended a national conference this year; role has current designated senior management responsibility; has demonstrated performance in current role.*

Step 2   *Invite staff to apply; address the criteria and state: reasons for requesting to attend; personal objectives for learning; strategy for dissemination of information upon return; detailed costing; resource arrangements in their area if necessary.*

Step 3   *Review applications with another staff member not immediately associated.*

Step 4   *Interview any staff if the information is unclear.*

These three examples show how situations can be analysed and how a suitable method of handling the situation can be implemented.

Methods using internal resources

Methods can be classified as unstructured or structured, referring more to planning rather than implementation. For example, an unplanned, un–structured discussion can still be implemented in a structured way, rather than in a haphazard way.

Unstructured

Such methods certainly appear more spontaneous and less planned. For example, you might be attending a staff meeting where the topic of replacement of staff during periods of leave is being discussed. Various comments are made and you note from the discussion that staff seem to express little respect or commitment towards the employer with statements like:

> I plan on taking my leave when I want to. The hospital can just cope the best it can.
> Why should I accommodate anyone else? No one considers me when they apply for leave.
> There's very little acknowledgment of a good job in this place. You are just expected to always give. When it comes to my leave, I intend to just take it.

It is not difficult to recognise that there is a problem being expressed here. Staff are feeling unappreciated and taken for granted. Attitudes such as those expressed do not indicate quality of work life. There may be an opportunity to explore the topic right then, or the issue may need to be discussed and dealt with later. If discussion can occur, some open questioning and rephrasing may be useful. For example:

> I am hearing quite a lot of frustration and anger in some people's statements. If I am right, I think we should talk about this further. (to statement #1)
> In what way do you think you receive an indication of your performance in your job? (to statement #2)
> Has anyone had to change their leave request because it clashed with someone else's, and if so, how did that feel? (to statement #3)

Here are some examples of where unstructured methods or techniques might be appropriate.

Example 1: At the completion of an interview and selection process, one of the participants says: *I had some difficulty making a decision here. I feel I didn't have sufficient information. How could that be improved in the future?*

The discussion that follows might result in:

- a review of selection criteria
- rewording of questions
- selection of different personnel on the panel
- a review of the documentation/evidence required.

Example 2: A death occurs in the operating suite during a very full day of cases. Staff are obviously upset but are too busy on the day to take time to review the situation and de-brief. The next day, the atmosphere is very tense and staff who were at work yesterday are obviously experiencing symptoms of stress. The manager identifies the need to intervene fairly quickly and to implement some way to address the situation. The manager makes some changes to staff allocation and arranges for those involved to have lunch at the same time. All staff are told why the changes have been made and those involved are invited to identify how they would like the situation to be handled, immediately and in the future. From this brief but focused discussion a number of strategies are planned. An immediate de-briefing session can occur and a program for all staff on coping with unexpected death is arranged.

Example 3: Following a considerable period of support and ongoing appraisal, the performance of a staff member is considered unsatisfactory and the staff member is given notice that the employment is to be terminated. The process of bringing this to fruition includes an exit interview at the end of which you feel satisfied with the evidence and action, but quite uncomfortable. You express your feelings to your manager who suggests you give all the relevant information to him/her to review and then convene a meeting to discuss the situation. In the meantime you make inquiries of other staff who had similar situations to deal with and try to compare your behaviour with theirs. At the end of the process, you feel you have a better understanding of the situation and that you handled the matter well.

What are the common threads in these three examples?

- There is an openness to learning.
- There is a desire to recognise and make the most of situations, regardless of the discomfort at the time.
- There is a commitment to development.
- The situations were not planned (structured) but the action that resulted certainly had structure to it.

Structured

There are many structured methods or techniques, many of which are most commonly used during the orientation-consolidation-continuing education phase of the staff development process. All of the methods could, however, be used at any time. The most common methods or techniques are discussed below showing how they may be applied.

Didactic

This method is often viewed as a lecture, or in the form of formal instruction referred to as teaching (I want to teach you something). It is a formal, carefully planned dissertation by someone who is seen to be knowledgeable on the topic. We have all experienced didactic presentations and almost any topic can be presented in this way. For example:

- a presentation to all new staff by the Chief Executive Officer on the mission and objectives of the organisation
- a lecture on evacuation methods or occupational health and safety protocols
- an after dinner speaker at a staff social function
- a key note speaker at a conference.

Didactic presentations have some recognisable characteristics.

Characteristics of didactic presentations

Suitable for audiences of any size
Can be informative (lecture), entertaining (speech) or rousing (rally)
The audience role is predominantly passive
Information flows one way
Feedback for the speaker is limited
Success depends on the knowledge and presentation skills of the speaker
Require specific facilities such as good seating, visual aids, public address system, raised platform

If you are intending to present a lecture or speech, the following guidelines will be useful:

Guidelines for presenting a lecture or speech

Know your topic and prepare well in advance.
Refer to your notes but avoid long periods of reading, unless that is asked for.
Make frequent eye contact with the audience
Use visual aids to support your material.
Review and summarise throughout and at the end.
Avoid the urge to include too much information, which will overload the audience.
Use handouts only to emphasise key points or to summarise.
Use humour if you are comfortable with it, but avoid it if you are not sure.
Make sure the equipment is ready and working before you commence.
Start and finish with a key statement, or something controversial, to establish attention.

It is worth noting that audience participation can be achieved with this type of presentation by asking questions, or inviting an indication of agreement by a show of hands. You can pause and get participants to stand and stretch, to talk to the person sitting next to them. With experience, you will learn to read your audience and to know when they are with you and interested, and when you have lost their attention. There are times when this method may be the best choice for the situation, the audience, the time frame or the topic. There are also times when other choices should be considered.

Meetings

Meetings can also be a useful structured method of dealing with a staff development situation. The number of meetings that must be attended is often a source of considerable irritation among staff, especially if they are poorly run, have no clear purpose and achieve no action. Any gathering together of people should, however, be viewed as a possible opportunity for staff development. The characteristics of a good meeting (Hayes 1988) are identified here:

Characteristics of a good meeting

- Establish a good reason for convening the meeting and question whether there is a better way to address the matter.
- Develop an agenda that is realistic.
- Advise participants of the details of the meeting, including the purpose, agenda and preparation necessary at least ten days in advance. Avoid rushed meetings.
- Start and end on time. Be ruthless as the chairperson and keep to the time frame. Defer items if necessary and cut off discussion.
- Aim for consensus decisions but allow individuals to express opinions and to differ.
- Encourage useful debate when appropriate.
- Be prepared to deal with difficult situations characterised by interpersonal conflict; that is, someone trying to dominate, someone who wants to argue, someone who meets with the neighbour rather than participating, someone who is negative and/or sceptical.
- Ensure accurate, concise minutes are distributed promptly to participants.

If the discussion is open, informed and purposeful, many opportunities may arise where a staff development issue/situation can be addressed effectively.

Interactive

The methods described here represent those where learning is most likely to occur because the participants are more involved in the learning process. Such methods include workshops, peer learning using a preceptor, demonstration, and role play. All methods call for facilitation although some presentation does occur. Some examples of staff development activities most suitable for interactive methods:

- *Workshop* on creative ways to manage stressful situations in the work place
- *Preceptor* learning for new nursing graduates
- *Demonstration* of clinical techniques in a laboratory situation
- *Peer teaching* of the administration of medications for new staff as part of their orientation program
- *Role play* to learn effective interviewing, debriefing, counselling and/or assertive communication skills.

A number of criteria can be recognised:

- Numbers are restricted as the most effective learning occurs with personal interaction.
- Learning is individual, meaningful and more likely to be internalised, therefore more likely to result in behaviour change.

163

- An experienced facilitator is required, with confidence in the subject area and well developed interpersonal skills.
- The interaction is rewarding for both presenter and participants.
- It is time consuming and resource intensive.

Many feel reluctant to use an interactive method or technique because of the criteria described above. It is easier to present the material without interaction or to facilitate a group discussion. The benefits are significant, however, and an opportunity to use one of these methods should be grasped. If you are planning to use an interactive method, such as a workshop, the following guidelines may help:

Guidelines for an interactive method

- Plan well ahead, including venue, time, personnel, materials.
- Set clear objectives and remain focussed even though participants will often wander off on a tangent.
- Plan the session to allow for a short introduction or preamble, time for learning and time to review.
- Follow up on results and obtain feedback from participants.

These examples demonstrate how different methods requiring some interaction can be used:

Example 1: A panel *discussion* on the legal need for accurate documentation in nursing. Panel members include a medico-lawyer, senior management, practising nurses and doctor or administrator.

Example 2: A *hypothetical* on coronial inquiries following a sudden death in the operating suite, co-ordinated by a solicitor with experience in such matters. Participants include perioperative nursing staff, anaesthetist, surgeon, lawyer and investigating staff from the coronial office.

Example 3: A *discussion* between staff on a ward to develop protocols for performance appraisal procedures. The session may begin with a presentation of common protocols and then open up for discussion to encourage staff to express problems, concerns and ideas.

The use of teleconference, interactive workshops, preceptorship and mentors are some of the methods that deserve further discussion:

Teleconference

There may be situations when it is necessary to speak with a number of people who are in the same organisation, but different departments; or who are located in different suburbs, towns or even states. The phone provides a cost effective way to link people together for a short period of time. A teleconference can occur by simply linking people on a conference call facility of the telephone. In this situation, everyone can hear what is said and can participate in the conversation. A teleconference can also occur between individuals who are far apart. In this case, individuals can hear everything that is said, but must take turns to speak. Examples of situations suitable for either a conference call or teleconference are outlined.

Example 1: A new policy is disseminated to all participants before a call is made, requesting review, analysis, the identification of difficulties and recommendations. Regional managers are linked by phone by appointment and each participant is invited to comment. Notes are taken and disseminated to participants with amendments to the policy.

Example 2: Departmental managers are linked by phone by appointment and asked to comment on selection criteria for a new position soon to be advertised. From the discussion it is evident that there is considerable variation in expertise and understanding of selection criteria and so a face-to-face session is arranged.

Example 3: Individual staff are completing a self-directed learning package on practice implications associated with IV drug administration by nurses. Part of the learning is a teleconference between a group of learners during which they discuss the issues and the strategies they are suggesting to overcome these issues.

Teleconferences require careful planning and there are a few useful guidelines to maximise their effectiveness.

Guidelines for a teleconference

- Set clear, specific objectives.
- Send out pre-reading well in advance with guidelines for procedure, the discussion and instructions on the procedure.
- Introduce yourself and each participant, clarify the purpose and speak again to each participant at the conclusion of the conference.
- Explain that only one person can speak at a time, but that everyone will get a turn, and encourage people to take notes and to record any questions they have.
- Avoid getting bogged down—defer items, promise to follow up, send information later.
- Speak slowly, clearly and consistently.
- Refer to individuals by name and 'circulate' between them, making sure all participate.
- Ask questions to establish understanding.
- Follow up an individual if there appears to be a problem, or an individual need.
- Summarise the outcomes of the conference at the end, inviting participants to contact you if necessary.

Workshop

Workshop, by its title, means people will interact, work will be done and learning will occur through the method and the content. Although some individuals will come to an interactive workshop with some apprehension and even a little fear, interactive learning is enjoyable and can be a great deal of fun. Experience has shown me that any group can be facilitated to learn, providing the presenter is prepared to be enthusiastic, creative, light hearted, knowledgeable and a bit of an extrovert. There are a few guidelines to ensure maximum likelihood of success:

- Choose the venue carefully: open, airy, comfortable rooms are best; hire excellent equipment; use chairs but not tables unless required; flat, not tiered flooring.
- Plan the session carefully so material is presented in chunks, mixing content and method.
- Move people around frequently: never let them sit for too long.
- Use a variety of equipment, such as overhead projector, white board, music, props, workbooks or summary sheets.
- Prepare participants beforehand; suggest comfortable clothing, pre-reading if necessary.
- Create the group in the first ten minutes with an activity of maximum interaction, fun, minimum effort; activities are called 'icebreakers' or 'games'.
- Be clear about your objectives and realistic about the depth and breadth of information that can be presented.
- Aim to capture the preferred learning style of all participants at least some of the time (see Chapter 3).

Preceptorship

A preceptor is required to have more knowledge and experience than the learner, so it is inevitable that some learning will occur. The relationship may have been established for a specific purpose or situation, but once it develops it is not unusual to see learning occur in a number of areas. There is an element of supervision, evaluation, monitoring and teaching in a preceptor relationship. Preceptors are frequently used in clinical nursing situations where competence and confidence are being developed. It can also work where new staff are learning their role; for example, a developing manager. A less formal application of preceptorship may result in the development of the role of a *mentor*.

A mentor can be a teacher, a peer or colleague, a supervisor, an advanced practitioner—almost anyone committed to the development of someone's career to offer something to suit everyone (Vance 1994). When asked, an individual may identify one person who has had a significant impact on their career and may refer to them as a mentor. The relationship and the interaction can be informal and over a long period of time, but when interaction does occur it can be quite formal. A mentor might provide career advice and guidance, professional role modelling, intellectual stimulation, inspiration, teaching, advice, nurturance and/or emotional support. Individuals tend to select their own mentor through an experience, someone they found they could talk to or who helped them in a situation. Mentoring relationships can empower and inspire to assist people to realise their potential and to encourage people to seek opportunities and perhaps take risks (See also Ch. 3).

Demonstration

The *demonstration* of a clinical procedure is an integral part of nursing education and practice, as it is in other health professions. Demonstration brings theoretical learning to life and can occur in a controlled environment, like a laboratory; on a ward as part of a planned experience; or spontaneously because the opportunity arose. Demonstration is an opportunity to use every clinical situation as a possible learning/teaching situation. Demonstration may aim to teach a new task, introduce a new technique, reinforce a point or illustrate or dramatise a situation.

Preparation is essential, even when the demonstration has not been planned. It should include the collection of necessary equipment, practice, explanation, audience participation and return demonstration at least to some degree. Demonstration facilitates the internalisation of knowledge and skill, since trying for oneself is a powerful aid to learning. Having to demonstrate really ensures your own level of understanding. Practice is the key to success and should be accompanied by support and feedback.

Example 1: Arrangements are made on a ward to demonstrate a new clinical procedure to staff. Staff are then given the opportunity to practise the procedure under supervision and eventually to demonstrate competence.

Example 2: Following a number of incidents of back strain which have been reported to management, it is decided to arrange a demonstration of correct lifting techniques to staff. Staff are gathered together in small groups to watch and practise on each other, after which they are asked to demonstrate the correct technique.

Example 3: Cleaning staff report to their manager that they are having difficulty with the new floor polishers. They are heavy and awkward to manoeuvre. The staff feel concerned that they are going to develop injuries. A demonstration by the supplier is arranged for all cleaning staff at which they observe the correct procedure, have an opportunity to try using the polisher under supervision and to learn the best way to handle it. Eventually they are required to demonstrate their ability in the work place. The problem is resolved.

Role play

Role play (drama spot) allows for a real-life situation to be improvised and acted out in front of a group with or without a script. The group then discuss the implications of the performance for the situation under consideration.

Role play can be used to examine a human relationship problem or situation; search for solutions to an emotion-laden situation; provide insight into different attitudes; practise new skills. There are many advantages to the technique of role play:

- Stimulates discussion to resolve a problem.
- Allows for the adoption of behaviours other than our own to achieve a better understanding.
- Avoids real-life dangers of a trial-and-error approach.
- Adds drama and fun to learning.
- Breaks down barriers to communication.

Some people, of course, feel too timid or self conscious to act a role effectively. Role play does require some specific planning for it to be successful, at least in the initial stages. However, with practice participants can become skilled at taking on a role with little preparation. Planning should include measures to:

- Select actors carefully at least in the initial stages.
- Allow for improvisation as this encourages creativity and improves the performance.
- Prepare prompts and scenarios that are realistic, simple and meaningful to the group.
- Be aware of the possible need to de-brief people out of role if situations become intense and players become very involved.
- Present realistic expectations of performance, emphasising contribution rather than performance.

Example 1: Setting up an opportunity to role play through interview scenarios can be a very useful way of developing skills, where participants get an opportunity to be the interviewer and to be interviewed.

Example 2: Providing the opportunity for staff to role play client education situations can assist with both the understanding of the material and the presentation skill. Again, staff benefit from playing both the client and the staff member and challenging each other with difficult questions and poor understanding.

Example 3: Following the death of a client, a nurse expresses concern that he/she did not handle the situation with the family well. This nurse is very experienced and has handled similar situations capably on many occasions. You suggest that you role play the conversation with the family, with you taking the role of the family member. You ask the nurse to go through the scene just as before. You find that the nurse does handle the situation well, but the opportunity to go through it again causes the nurse to become emotional. With support and encouragement, he/she identifies some unresolved grief from a similar personal situation with a family member. This particular client reminded the nurse of that family member. The role play allows the nurse to recognise what had happened and to begin to work through unresolved feelings.

Self-directed

Self-directed methods of achieving staff development outcomes are becoming more popular as they can demonstrate efficient use of resources and because they represent a method that is particularly attractive to adult learners. Learners complete educational activities on their own, taking over the traditional educational task of a teacher. The learner takes control of their own learning by selecting, relating, analysing, structuring, personalising, memorising and rehearsing their learning. This type of learning process involves self observation, self judgement and self reflection. Self-directed methods and techniques are referred to as self-regulated, autonomous, independent study and self-organised study. Self-directed methods and techniques are built upon a number of education beliefs:

- Self-directed adults will retain and make better use of learning, than reactive learners.
- Effective adult life requires lifelong, continuous, effective, creative, self-guided learning, all of which are evident in self-directed learning.
- Motivation, attitudes, inner resources and skills needed to engage in this life long learning can be developed and enhanced by participating in well designed learning situations.
- Control of learning empowers individuals to take control of their life.

Self-directed learning methods have a number of specific characteristics:

- clearly defined goals for learning
- readily available resources
- competent facilitators
- administrative monitoring mechanisms
- a collaborative, not dependent, relationship between provider and learner
- understanding of the role and responsibilities of the provider and learner.

From these characteristics the following advantages become obvious:

- Learning is individualised and needs specific.
- Learners are able to identify exactly what they want to learn.
- Learners can achieve a determined level of competence.
- Progress is self-paced.
- Personal satisfaction of the learner is increased.
- Learners feel empowered and in control.
- Material is consistent and not subject to teacher variation.
- Time is used effectively.
- Resources can be reused and are cost effective.
- An alternative to traditional methods is provided.

There are of course also some disadvantages.

- Individuals are not necessarily used to this method; they may take time to adjust to the lack of direction and structure.
- The role of the teacher becomes much less personalised.

169

- There is an increased potential for dishonest behaviour as the system relies on trust.
- The onus for learning relies on the individual, which may not be appropriate or productive for that learner.

The success of a self-directed method depends on belief in the system, support of the principles of adult learning, confident and experienced teachers who do not seek to control the situation (who let go their control) and a commitment to considerable development of material in the initial stage. The process of development (Miller 1989) is quite specific:

Developing self-directed learning materials

- Select an appropriate topic with opportunity for repetition; cognitive and psychomotor topics (with demonstration) are both suitable.
- Consider the target audience; this decides the language and content.
- Identify the overall goal.
- Identify the learning objectives and outcome expectations.
- Develop the content; include an introduction or overview of the content and the process.
- Establish the style: conversational, one-to-one.
- Choose the instructional design: the artwork, written or on computer disk, using slides and/or audio tapes and/or video tapes, using pre-tests.
- Incorporate a practice cycle: small sequential steps, immediate feedback, questions and answers.
- Develop the evaluation instrument based upon scenarios or case studies, multiple choice and short answer tests.
- Pilot test the package.
- Establish the administrative mechanisms: access, availability, records
- Review annually and modify as necessary.

Because of the increasing interest in self-directed learning methods and techniques, many models can be found and some of the more common models will be discussed below.

Problem-based learning

Problem-based learning methods are a most effective method of learning and can be developed into a number of different types of learning packages. For example, to practise nursing effectively it is recognised that there is a need to integrate knowledge from a number of sources; theory, experience, practice and reflection. Many individuals need assistance to integrate knowing what and knowing how and this is more likely to occur within a problem-based approach to learning. Problem-based learning places the learner at the centre of the process of working towards the understanding or resolution of a problem. The learner becomes committed to critical reflection on clinical practice to create personal meaning and to challenge practices. The learner becomes the creator of knowledge rather than the receptor (Barrows in Crowe 1994).

Problem-based learning can be applied within almost any learning strategy. It is more likely to be effective however if learners are left alone to manage their own learning and encouraged to find out the answer. The application of this method can be seen in these examples:

Example 1: A problem-based orientation program to a ward where the individual has to find resources and answers through a series of hypothetical scenarios. The individual works through the scenarios by solving each problem as it is presented to them, learning about the environment as they find the solutions to the problems.

Example 2: A program on the triage and nursing management of casualty clients when they first arrive in the department, where each client is presented as a new problem and the learner has to work through the process of assessment, diagnosis, planning, action and outcome to learn the most appropriate case management. Cases are then presented to peers for feedback and confirmation.

A common problem-based learning approach involves the use of a case study presentation. A *case study* is an extensive description and analysis of a situation, group, or community presented in a real-life situation. A single case study looks at one situation with the intent of examining the relationship of the multiple variables, whereas a cross case study synthesises the lessons learnt from a number of cases for the purpose of developing generalised explanations. There are some limitations to case studies: they are time consuming, require multiple cognitive skills, are narrative based and may be extensive. They gather a great deal of information and sometimes run the risk of missing the truly significant points because of the quantity of data.

Case studies can be used to present a realistic situation where you may wish to demonstrate a particular aspect of learning:

Presenting an example of a work situation
A staff member gives notice unexpectedly and with no warning, leaving the area short staffed. You have to work through the options that are available to you. You need to reorganise the work load of remaining staff to maintain client care without compromising standards or placing remaining staff under undue pressure.

Teaching the importance of thorough assessment
Mr Jones presents as disinterested and depressed about his treatment but you cannot identify the cause of his depression. With thorough assessment and careful questioning, you identify that he has a number of other personal and social problems that are distracting him, all of which need to be addressed before he can focus on his treatment.

**Demonstrating the importance of having an open mind
and looking at the whole situation**

*Miss Brown is sixteen and pregnant and she presents at the hospital in
labour, alone, but in control and apparently very well prepared. The first
reaction of staff is to question her ability to care for this baby because of
her age. She is not easy to talk to and you have to work hard to find out
about her situation, so you can provide the most appropriate information
and support. As you work with her through her labour, you realise that
this young lady is very capable, well prepared and committed to her new
baby. The initial concern is unfounded.*

The advantages of this approach are the presentation of meaningful
situations (learners can relate to the situation), relevance to detail (missed
detail may change the solution), the identification of alternative solutions to
situations and the development of analytical skills (different options are
presented).

As in all areas of education, computers often open up all sorts of possibilities.
Computer assisted learning is becoming increasingly popular. Many specific skills
can be learnt through a computer software program; for example, word
processing, data base application. Computers can also be used to *assist* learning
through the use of interactive case studies that accompany a written topic; or
to *manage* the learning system within the testing process (multiple choice
questions, short answer questions and essay questions can all be written into
an exam, to be accessed by the learner) and to keep records. Individuals don't
have to be experts in word processing to gain the advantages of computer
assisted learning as the instructions are built within the program. Similarly,
the use of the material for testing is completed with a few key stokes through
a simple user-menu method of instruction.

Computer hardware is of course necessary. This can be expensive and
most organisations would look to establish a central laboratory or facility to
allow access by as many staff as possible. Materials could be made available to
staff to use in their own time on their own personal computers if that was the
agreed procedure. Here are some examples of how learning can be assisted by
a computer, with a self-directed learning package that uses an interactive case
study on disk, or a testing mechanism that allows access to a test bank of
questions.

Example 1: A self-directed learning package on clinical research consisting of
a workbook, readings and an interactive case study on disk, that shows the
learner how to go about clinical research (Southern Cross University, Lismore
NSW, Centre for Professional Development).

Example 2: A continuing education module (topic) titled, 'HIV Infection for
nurses' consisting of a self-directed workbook with readings, assessment by
multiple choice and short answer questions from within an established question
bank, which can be accessed by learners when they are ready to assess their

learning. When instructed, the test is printed, learners answer the questions, then enter their answers. The test is marked instantly, the result calculated and printed. Learners then know whether they can move on to the next topic or, following review, resit this topic at a later date and with a different test. This topic is part of a package of topics which form a nursing education program that is available for renewal of registration, migrant bridging education and continuing education (Curtin University of Technology School of Nursing, WA).

Example 3: A common clinical topic such as breast self examination is developed into an interactive computer program for distance learning purposes. It is based on a case study of a woman who presents to a remote nursing clinic for a regular health check and it is suspected that she has a breast lump. The program teaches the nurse how to complete a thorough assessment, including techniques and health teaching. The learner works through the program making decisions about the best way to conduct the examination and offer the best health information for the woman in that situation. The program takes the nurse through initial questioning, assessment and diagnosis, health teaching and follow-up, dealing with personal, family and social pressures and problems.

Many academic institutions are using computers to assist learning within courses and it is only a matter of time before they are in common use in health care organisations.

Train-the-trainer

A discussion on methods would be incomplete without reference to train-the-trainer programs. For many educators, myself included, the term train-the-trainer sits uncomfortably with principles of learning and teaching. Education occurs when an individual is assisted and supported to learn, where the learning is entirely in their control. Training, on the other hand, is the acquisition of knowledge and skill as directed by the trainer. The process and the outcomes are quite different. Therefore, when you train someone to be able to train individuals, you give them the knowledge and skills to be able to do what you just did, but education did not necessarily occur.

There is certainly a place for training in the work place. Expertise can be taught very successfully and competence can be demonstrated. It is, however, the acquisition of specific expertise for a given situation and/or task. It is not always transferable. It tends to be a discrete, specific, short term solution, and for that it is very successful. Certainly others can be trained to train in this way. But it is a far less complex level of learning and not always appropriate for some aspects of staff development, where the process should focus on the facilitation of education and aim to empower individuals to want to learn for themselves. Knowledge and skill are then internalised and are transferable. You can see the results of training; you cannot always see the results of education.

Unfortunately, as money for staff development has decreased with the call for cost effectiveness and the number of staff with staff development positions decrease, train-the-trainer programs are being viewed as a way to increase the number of individuals who can teach and are considered a viable alternative to (specialist) education. In terms of long term outcomes, the effectiveness has not been demonstrated. It is of concern when academic institutions, where there is suppose to be a commitment to the philosophy, principles and practices of education, market train-the-trainer programs for teachers, to train teachers how to train new teachers. The same concern has arisen with tertiary and community programs that teach tasks to individuals to enable them to work in the health sector as un-registered, unqualified health workers.

A train-the-trainer program should be planned, implemented and evaluated in the same rigorous manner as any other learning. There are no acceptable short cuts (Zaccarelli H E 1988). It is likely that the objectives would be less complex, the content have less depth, the expected outcomes more specific and the presentation would certainly be more teacher centred. Training people to train others has the potential to meet the operational needs of an organisation, at least in the short term, but not necessarily to put into place the foundations for long term development and growth.

Methods using external resources

The methods discussed in this section are grouped together because they all use resources outside the organisation. They are not initiated by the organisation. Using external methods can be particularly cost effective and resource efficient particularly for smaller organisations or ones with a very specific or narrow focus.

Short courses

Providers, such as tertiary institutions, training companies, professional organisations and government authorities, offer short courses in topics ranging from computer skills to retirement planning and management models. They can focus on interpersonal skill development (conflict resolution, effective communication, team building), on specific job related skills (word processing, skills audits, epidural analgesia, budget management), or on increasing knowledge (workers compensation legislation, customer charters, management of clients with HIV/AIDS). There is no limit to the topics that can be presented as a short course. Participants expect to receive a certificate of attendance/ achievement and the topic is usually quite specific, often necessarily narrow in its focus, but quite intensive.

Characteristics of short courses are identified as:

- off site attendance; participants are not necessarily from the same organisation; courses can be brought into the organisation specifically for staff

- planned and advertised well in advance and marketed competitively
- structured in presentation but not restricted to traditional learning and teaching methods
- cost, content and presenter are predetermined
- clearly identified as a learning activity and therefore participants are removed from every day work routine
- expectations of outcomes are often unrealistic as courses are standardised and not individually needs based
- numbers usually limited
- if not organisation specific, difficult to evaluate effectiveness or outcomes as participants often come from a range of backgrounds and organisations
- groups heterogeneous and individuals are not necessarily at the same level of knowledge and skill; presentation tends to be to the group not to individuals
- require a financial and time commitment.

Attendance at short courses is often initiated by the individual but the organisation may seek out a course for an individual in response to specific need. Obviously, if the organisation is meeting the costs of the course, they will expect the individual to gain benefit and to see evidence for their investment. Short courses can be offered by traditional methods involving face-to-face presentation and therefore, attendance, or by distance delivery and a self-directed approach.

Example 1: A short course on *Effective Communication* is advertised by the Australian Institute of Management, involving attendance for four half days over a period of two weeks. The course is held at the office of the Institute and at a set price. The content is set and there is no opportunity to modify the content to individual need. Participants come from a range of organisations. The health care organisation chooses to send a manager who has identified, during performance appraisal, a need to develop his/her communication skills.

Example 2: A computer training company offers a course called *Introduction to Word processing.* The course runs all day for three consecutive days at the training venue of the company, where hardware is available. The course includes a workbook and exercises to practice newly developed skills, back at work. The numbers are limited to fifteen because of equipment, the cost is set and the organisation chooses to send all clerical staff with word processing responsibilities, over a period of months.

Example 3: A University School of Nursing offers a number of clinical related topics by distance education, as self-directed learning packages, as part of their continuing education initiatives. Individuals pay by module and use the library and other resources of the University. Successful completion of a topic results in a certificate. If individuals choose to enrol in formal studies later as part of an award course, they can apply for credit towards a specific unit within the degree course. Individuals at this organisation enrol of their own initiative.

Conferences and conventions

From any journal or newsletter it is easy to identify at least two conferences each year that you would like to attend. The range of topics and locations are endless. Every professional organisation, most academic institutions and many government departments, seem to offer annual or bi-annual conferences. Topics are usually presented as a broad theme to allow presentation on a range of related issues, usually over one to three days. Because of the number of conferences offered, competition is fierce, and, unfortunately, topics often overlap both within and between conferences. How can you select a good conference either as an individual wishing to attend, or as an organisation choosing to send staff as part of a staff development program? After many years of personal experience as a convenor, presenter and participant, I believe there are a number of essential features. These may assist you to choose a conference and/or be useful if you find yourself involved in planning or convening one, a practice that is becoming more common in forward thinking organisations.

Features of a good conference for delegates or convenors

- clear, meaningful theme with titles for sessions that explain the breadth and depth of the subject area without jargon
- program that is comprehensive but not crowded and which includes breaks and opportunities for networking and mixing
- quality venue with all facilities available and functional
- capable efficient management of the program, content, venue, activities and administration; particularly important as a convenor
- program that offers a range of informative, innovative, challenging, futuristic and controversial presentations over a wide range of topics
- mixture of presentation styles to offer something to suit everyone: plenary (key note and major presentations), concurrent (offered at the same time), interactive and informal
- presenters who are chosen for the expertise and their presentation skills
- quality publications that include at least a program, abstracts and synopsis of the presentations and presenters, and usually a book of proceedings available at the end of the conference
- evaluation strategies during the conference and follow up after. As a participant it is important to give feedback, and, as a convenor it is essential to receive feedback
- information about a range of convenient accommodation options and travel, if necessary.

Conferences and conventions usually have a significant cost and value for money is absolutely essential. Conventions may offer a less comprehensive program and follow a more traditional presentation style than a conference.

Conventions are often associated more with regional sub-groups of an organisation while conferences bring together a wide range of individuals.

Individuals may request to attend a conference or convention for its specific relevance and their specific interest/need. Or an employer may seek out an individual to attend for their or the organisation's need or relevance, or because the organisation needs to be seen/represented. Regardless of the reason for attending, a report or feedback strategy should be implemented. It is valuable experience to be a presenter at a conference and individuals benefit from being encouraged to consider making a contribution through a paper, poster display, or information stand. Involvement tends to raise the motivation for learning even though guidance may be required to develop a presentation. Assistance may be needed in any or all of these areas: to write an abstract, write a paper, develop a poster display, chair a meeting or session, set up an information stand or convene a special interest group. Certainly individuals may feel apprehensive at first, but with the right guidance it can be a great learning experience.

Seminars

A seminar usually involves convening a group to study a topic in depth under the guidance of a recognised expert. The topic is usually quite specific; for example, the re-use of single use items in surgery, the implementation of casemix management, funder/provider services, or current developments in clinical management of juvenile arthritis. A well run seminar will include detailed and systematic discussion. Seminars usually require some pre-reading or research and participants must come prepared to contribute and be involved. The expert must have recognised knowledge and expertise and have credibility with the group. Seminars need to be co-ordinated well as the co-ordinator will be required to keep the participants on track while encouraging inquiry, discussion and debate.

Because the topic tends to be more specific it may be recognised as more employment specific and more attractive to an employer. Cost is usually not prohibitive as the seminar is usually presented locally or close by to facilitate attendance by interested local parties. A clear statement of the topic is essential as is a statement of objectives and expected outcomes to assist participants and presenters to focus. All of the requirements of a good learning environment apply; that is, appropriate facilities, equipment, comfort, refreshments and timing. Evaluation and feedback from participants are also very beneficial, and a follow-up with participants encouraged.

Visits, tours and secondments

These options are all characterised by a planned itinerary, during which an environment, past or present activity, or position can be studied. Unfortunately, this method is frequently viewed, at its simplest level, as being too informal to be credible; or, at its most complex level, as too difficult. Organisations are often pleased to show off a practice that has been recognised as successful and usually very willing to share information and/or expertise. They may one day wish to seek the same from another organisation.

Seeing is always more meaningful than hearing or reading alone and it then becomes easier to apply. Far more can be learnt by observing something actually working in an environment than from hearing about it from someone else. Obviously, there is need for careful planning and a mutual agreement to ensure a successful outcome. How might this work? At the simplest level, a manager may identify a need to examine different methods of a specific clinical procedure. Following inquiry, it is identified that three other organisations are using this method slightly differently, all with successful outcomes. All organisations indicate agreement to a visit by two relevant staff. The manager chooses the staff, both of whom are knowledgeable in the procedure and who indicate a desire to implement the new method. Following discussion the purpose of the visit is identified, specific objectives are set and agreement is reached on a reporting mechanism that will gather and analyse the data. Formal contact is made with the three organisations advising them of the objectives of the visit, suggesting activities, an introduction to the people involved and a proposed time frame. The arrangements are successful and the visits go ahead.

At a more complex level, organisation A is planning a major restructuring of its management structure and practices. The planning committee are working on the stage where staff are advised of the proposed changes and given an opportunity to question and comment. A member of the group explains that a particular organisation he/she had previously worked in (organisation B) had completed a similar exercise with great success in the past and were in the process of repeating this technique again in another area. Following negotiation it is arranged to send the chairperson of the planning group and one other member to work in organisation B for a month to actively observe the method and its impact on the employees. In exchange, organisation B requests to send an employee to organisation A to work in Intensive Care to experience the client case management model that is in place and which has proven to be so effective. Certainly, this involves more formal negotiations and consideration of employment conditions and other matters, but there are benefits for both organisations and it is a relatively simple application of a staff development method.

Planning for presentation

Regardless of the method, the time comes to act and potential successes can be turned to disaster for lack of attention to the details of the presentation. Presentation in this context refers to the actual performance of the individual as well as the preparation and use of equipment and materials. It is indeed the little things that make the difference, and planning is essential. Some aspects of presentation have already been discussed when discussing an individual method, so these comments are presented in a general way and can be viewed as helpful hints or guidelines to maximise success.

Venues

When choosing a venue consider and rate the following:

1 Quality of service
 —quality of catering
 —timing of catering
 —provision of equipment
 —maintenance of equipment
 —attendance to setting up rooms/equipment
 —attendance to messages, phones, fax
2 Quality of equipment
3 Rooms
 —size, shape, access, lighting
4 Aesthetics/levels of comfort
5 Distractions and noise
6 Resources and equipment
7 Overall costing: base and peripherals
8 Flexibility with equipment.

Equipment and materials

The following diagram demonstrates the value of various aids to learning and serves as a guide when choosing equipment and materials (Moss 1987).

The selection of equipment can also be guided by determining the primary purpose, because each method, with its strengths and weaknesses, may call for specific materials (Moss 1987).

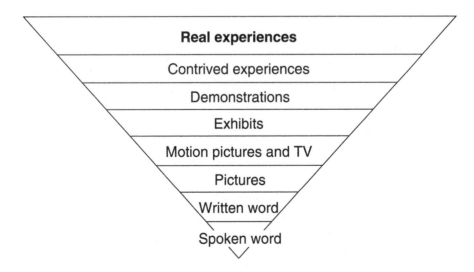

Fig. 7.1 Relative value of aids to learning

Primary purpose

To transfer knowledge, use:
    group discussion; questions and answers
    group exercise or activity
    lectures, with handouts
    panel discussions
    audio visual material: films, videos
To practise problem solving, use:
    case studies
    brain-storming
    discussion groups
To develop skills, use:
    demonstration for manual skills
    role playing, for interpersonal skills
    peer teaching
    programmed instruction
To change attitudes, use:
    debates
    visual displays
    role playing, for revealing how others feel
    group discussion, for group attitudes
    individual projects
    demonstrations

Some equipment and materials have quite specific uses and this summary of common equipment and materials and their features forms a useful guide:

Equipment and materials

Printed materials supplement many other materials
    provide for review of information at learner's own pace
    may be individualised
    useful only with literate learners
    must be in language of reader
Whiteboards may be used in larger groups
    inexpensive
    re-useable
    may require advance preparation
    no way of preserving images (unless electronic)
Slides/films appropriate for individual, small group or large groups with instruction
    easily stored and revised
    present many images

Audio tapes	may be altered to meet individual needs
	need specific equipment
	must be good quality
	can be used for individual or group instruction
	prepared with inexpensive equipment
	economical to duplicate
	can be used alone or in conjunction with other materials
	fixed cost for information giving
	possible to erase messages
Overhead	permit eye contact between instructor and learner
transparencies	prepared and stored easily and inexpensively
	operated and maintained easily
	use to highlight, reinforce or supplement verbal instruction
	can be used repeatedly
	poor production is common
	text must be clear, brief and large
Videos	appropriate for individuals and groups
	provide realism
	portable
	minimise audience interaction
	benefit increases if guides for discussion are included
	expensive

Presentation

Presentation usually refers to the actual process of delivering material, during a lecture, talk or speech, but it is just as important in a meeting, interview, discussion or demonstration. Presentation is about your personal performance, how you come across to your audience. A good beginning is to examine your own behaviour and identify which category best describes you (Mandel 1987).

Category	*Characteristic*
Avoider	An avoider does everything possible to escape from having to get in front of an audience. In some cases avoiders may seek positions that do not call for making presentations at all.
Resister	A resister has fear when asked to speak. This fear may be strong. Resisters may not be able to avoid speaking as part of their job, but they never encourage it. When they do speak they do so with great reluctance and considerable pain.

Accepter	The accepter will give presentations as part of the job but does not seek those opportunities.
	Accepters occasionally give a presentation and feel like they did a good job. They even find that once in a while they are quite persuasive and enjoy speaking in front of a group.
Seeker	A seeker looks for opportunities to speak. The seeker understands that anxiety can be a stimulant which fuels enthusiasm during a presentation.
	Seekers work at building their professional communi-cation skills and self-confidence by speaking often.

Depending on your analysis, you will be able to see specific areas where you need to work on yourself. For example, if you are an *avoider* you need to seek out opportunities; if you are an *accepter* you need to move yourself outside your area of comfort and use your initiative to seek out new opportunities. Presentation is about making your message memorable and a message will be memorable if it is interesting, useful, credible, understandable, practical and considerate (Malouf 1988). If a presentation is about adopting new techniques or making changes, and most are to some degree, the technique requires motivation, attitude, support, and knowledge.

Motivation and attitude are under the control of the individual and the final decision remains with them. However the presentation can certainly have an influence on the listener. Too often learning is confused with knowledge only; unless the other components are present, change is unlikely.

Regardless of the method you are using, this checklist will assist you in your preparation and presentation.

- Inspect the venue.
- Check the equipment.
- Mix with the group before the presentation.
- Write your own introduction.
- Aim to make an impact in the first three minutes.
- Introduce your topic/purpose.
- Smile and be enthusiastic.
- Show you are interested in what you are presenting.
- Reinforce and repeat.
- Use examples and mnemonics to illustrate.
- Induce participation.
- Keep it moving.
- Summarise to close.
- End on a high note.

The following are labelled as the *deadly sins* for presenters (Pike 1993) :

- failure to keep to time; arrive late, start late, go over time
- appear unprepared; material not suitable for the audience, material not prepared, equipment not ready
- information overload; disregard for the learner/person's personal need
- botch the audiovisual; poor quality, poor handling, unsatisfactory equipment or placement
- fail to address the audience; avoid making eye contact, read everything
- handle question poorly; bluff your way through an answer, be afraid to admit you don't know, act aggressively and/or defensively to questions.

Finally, there is an art to effective presentation and the most effective presenters are larger than life, confident, attractive and humorous, as well as informative. There is an actor within every good presenter. Good presentation comes with practice which builds confidence and experience. At the beginning, accept your level of expertise and acknowledge that to feel anxious is healthy; indeed, some of that anxiety never goes, for anxiety is a natural state that exists any time you are placed in an unusual situation. Presenting, or speaking in public (1-100 people) will cause some anxiety. Physical symptoms of a nervous stomach, sweating, tremor, twitches, accelerated breathing and/or increased heart rate are all normal. The skill is to recycle that energy into a positive form, to get all the butterflies flying in one direction.

Tips to deal with anxiety

Organise: be prepared for your topic and audience
Visualise: see yourself as successful
Practice: each time will be better
Breathe: tightness and tension are related to oxygen deficiency
Focus on relaxing: practice physical and mental relaxation
Release the tension: use isometric exercise
Move: release muscle tension
Make eye contact with the audience: create a personal connection

Chapter summary

This chapter has discussed many different methods to achieve staff development outcomes. The principles behind the best choice for a situation should be, to obtain the maximum result, to have the greatest impact, and/or to bring about a behaviour change that is a result of growth and development. Methods were discussed in groups, first, methods using internal resources, and second, methods using external resources. Some situations lend themselves to particular methods and with experience, you will be able to select the most appropriate method for any situation. Regardless of which method you choose, the time comes for presentation. Aspects of presentation that were considered here were venues, equipment and materials, personal performance. There are no fixed rules when it comes to methods. Just consider all the relevant factors, be prepared to be innovative and creative and remember that your aim is always to achieve the best possible outcome.

REFERENCES

Crowe M 1994 Problem-based learning: a model for graduate transition in nursing. Contemporary Nurse 3(3):105-109

Hayes M 1988 Effective meeting skills: a practical guide for more productive meetings. Crisp Publications, Los Altos, California

Malouf D 1988 How to create and deliver a dynamic presentation. Simon Schuster, Australia

Mandel S 1987 Effective presentation skills: a practical guide for better speaking. Crisp Publications, Menlo Park, California

Miller P J 1989 Developing self-directed learning packages. Journal of Nursing Staff Development, March/April 73-77

Moss G 1987 The trainers handbook: for managers and trainers. Moss and Associates, New Zealand

Pike B 1993 Creative training concepts. T & D Focus, AITD March 15-16

Vance C 1994 Mentoring for career success and satisfaction. The Australian Journal of Advanced Nursing 11:4 3

Zaccarelli H E 1988 Training managers to train: a practical guide to improving employee performance. Crisp Publications, Los Altos, California

8

Skills for staff development

Key questions

- What personal qualities are necessary for effective performance in staff development?

- What essential behaviours are necessary for the staff development role?

- What conceptual skills are necessary for key performance?

- What are recommended qualifications and experience for staff development?

- How can the employer gain the most benefit from the staff development role?

Content summary

Introduction

Personal qualities for effective performance in staff development

Essential behaviours for the staff development role

Skills for staff development
    Human skills
    Technical skills
    Conceptual skills
        Recommended formal qualifications and experience
        Essential attributes

References

Introduction

There are no specific formal qualifications or experience that are essential for a role in staff development as there are for a role as a nurse or other health professional. The role is complex and difficult to define in terms of specific attributes because it can vary between organisations and professions. The role involves a number of activities, especially if there is a staff development process implemented within the organisation. All of the activities involve working with people, either directly or indirectly. It is a people-oriented role. It is possible however to identify the qualities necessary for effective performance in a staff development role, the essential behaviours for the role, and the skills to be successful in the role; and to suggest qualifications and experience for the role. Finally, an organisation can be guided to get the best results for their investment; that is, from the person employed in a staff development role.

Personal qualities for effective performance in staff development

Donovan and Jackson (1991) have identified a list of qualities necessary to carry out effective human resource management. As staff development includes the management of human resources, I have modified the list to represent the qualities I consider to be necessary for effective performance in a staff development role; that is, what do you as a person need to be able to do. They are discussed here, but in no particular order of importance.

It is necessary that a person in a staff development role is able to:

Plan. Planning involves establishing a balance between short term and long term goals. In a staff development role, you are continually setting, modifying and resetting goals to achieve both short term and long term outcomes.

Work with change. The role requires the ability to recognise where and when change is needed; to plan for change to occur; to implement and respond to change.

Balance needs. The role requires the ability to balance both individual and organisational needs; to identify needs; to resolve conflict between different needs; to deal with multiple needs.

Depersonalise situations. Because the role involves working with people, there is a call to remain detached, to remove yourself from situations and from individuals. You can give of yourself in situations, but should avoid adopting or taking on the emotions and personal problems/concerns of others.

Work consistently. As you are working within a process and also with many different groups and individuals, you should demonstrate consistency to yourself and to others.

Show commitment. The demands of the role make it necessary to be accepting of, and comfortable with, the ethos of the organisation and to be committed to your role within the organisation.

Communicate. Effective, sensitive, open communication is essential to the success of the role, in both written and verbal communication.

Self-criticise. Success depends on your ability to recognise your need for knowledge and skills, to evaluate your performance and outcomes and to acknowledge your achievements and success.

Facilitate. There is a significant role in facilitating the growth and development of others, which requires the giving and receiving of feedback through open honest communication.

Focus on process and outcome. In the staff development role the process is as important as the outcome; the process needs to be the most appropriate for each situation to achieve the required outcome.

Work independently and with others. The role requires the discipline and confidence to work alone as well as the ability to work with others.

Feel confident. The role sometimes places an individual either isolated from or in conflict with others, in terms of decisions that must be made; the role may make you feel isolated, both physically and personally.

Lead. The role requires the ability to influence others towards the achievement of goals, where the influence can come through ones own behaviour, attitude, opinion or through actions; leadership is often judged at times of stress or crises; this role also calls for leadership in routine situations and events.

Essential behaviours for the staff development role

The staff development role is concerned with achieving outcomes successfully with and through the efforts of others, and using resources effectively and efficiently. The staff development role requires considerable management expertise; that is, the ability to manage your role. Hunt (1986) describes three components to a management role:

- a relating role: to peers, colleagues, superiors
- an informational role: clarifying goals, informing, planning
- a decision role: allocating resources, resolving conflict, implementing action.

How well the individual performs within the role is often demonstrated through a very personalised work style/behaviour. However, it is this capacity to cope with the many behaviours of the role, that is, to think of many things at once, to shift rapidly from one activity to another, to think laterally, to see consequences before others do, that provides evidence of effective performance in the role. Key behaviours are described as broadly as possible here, recognising that there will be considerable variation between organisations. Again they are discussed in no particular order of importance.

Implement organisation aims and objectives

The staff development role is often perceived to be the action of the organisation, for it is through staff development activities that you can best see where the organisation is heading and how successful it is. The work involves considerable time implementing the aims and objectives of the organisation.

Develop personal values

There is a need to examine your own values particularly towards such things as education, growth and development, quality of work life, indicators of performance, and role expectations.

Establish targets

With such a range of activities, it is essential to set realistic targets with specific outcomes.

Organise and develop available human, material and financial resources to achieve outcomes

Organisation and development of human resources includes selection, orientation, appraisal, counselling, career planning, job design, and education.

Organisation of material resources includes purchasing, asset management, information technology, and learning resources.

Organisation of financial resources includes budgeting, fundraising, cost benefit analysis, costing, and marketing.

Control, monitor and evaluate processes and outcomes

The activities of the role are directed towards both the processes and the outcomes; as indicated earlier, each are equally important.

Establish standards of performance

Many of the activities of the role relate to the establishment of a standard, or as a result of an established standard not being achieved.

Implement change

Change may be implemented through any stages of the staff development process. The role requires the ability to focus on change for both employer and employee.

Recognise and respond to signs of negative stress

The role often places the individual in a position to recognise when things are not going well for either an individual or the organisation in general. It is not unusual for the staff development role to include activities for individuals such as debriefing, counselling, and the management of stress; or activities for the organisation such as recognising poor performance, receiving client complaints, and recognising failure to achieve required outcomes.

Having now examined the role in some detail, it is easier to identify and discuss the skills necessary for success in a staff development role.

Skills for staff development

Skills necessary for success in a staff development role can be broken down into three groups (Hunt 1986).

- human skills: interpersonal skills
- technical skills: decision and knowledge skills
- conceptual skills: planning and visionary skills

Each group is discussed with emphasis on those skills perceived to be most readily applied in health care organisations.

Human skills

All human skills involve some aspect of communication and in particular, listening skills. Individual skills are listed as goal setting, negotiating, self-management, motivating, facilitating, coaching, appraising, rewarding, team building, resolving conflict, leading, problem solving, and communicating. Those skills that are most readily applied are resolving conflict, motivating to learn, and self-management.

Resolving conflict

Resolving conflict is singled out for discussion because there are many aspects of the staff development role where there is the potential for conflict. Inevitably it is the person in staff development who becomes involved in resolving the conflict situation. Examples of conflict situations include: resolving conflict between individual and organisational goals; resolving conflict between individual staff members; resolving conflict between what is required by the organisation and what is preferred by staff. The ability to resolve conflict is most frequently seen within the counselling and appraising components of the role. Within any organisation there is conflict, however; conflict is not always negative. Conflict may give rise to emotions of anger and resentment and to unproductive behaviour/interaction. Conflict can be interpersonal, occurring between two or more people when attitudes, values and expectations are incompatible and individuals perceive they are in conflict. Conflict can also be intrapersonal, occurring within an individual when there are equally attractive options but only one must be chosen. Conflict can also be constructive and energise a relationship or interaction.

Destructive conflict can:

- prevent individuals from seeing the task at hand
- subvert overall objectives in favour of those of sub-groups
- lead people to use defensive and blocking behaviour
- result in disintegration of an entire group
- stimulate win-lose interaction where reason is secondary

On the other hand, constructive conflict can:

- introduce alternative solutions to a problem
- clearly define the power relationships within a group
- focus on individual contributions rather than group decisions
- provide a means of dealing with emotive, non-rational arguments in the open
- provide for catharsis: release of long standing conflict.

Conflict usually arises in relation to one of four areas: skills, knowledge, attitudes, or values. For example, conflict may arise when two people have different levels of skill and it has been assumed that the skill levels are the same. Conflict may arise when the knowledge within a group varies when it has been assumed that everybody has the same knowledge. Similarly, conflict can arise when individuals have different attitudes towards a situation or event. Finally, conflict can arise when individuals hold different values that they believe put them in conflict with each other. Conflict can be resolved. As much conflict has the potential to be constructive, the aim should be to use the conflict, to allow it to be exorcised and dealt with openly and so stimulate discussion and debate. Unfortunately, most conflict is not dealt with. Rather it is ignored and so little value can be obtained from the situation.

There are five common responses to conflict: withdraw, dominate, give in, attack or collaborate. If you *withdraw* (denial) you become less assertive, more controlled, hold in your feelings, keep quiet and fail to share your ideas. You avoid, dodge, escape and retreat from other people and/or undesirable situations. If you *dominate* (power) you tend to become over assertive, autocratic, unbending and over controlling, demanding that things be done your way. You have a very strong will and attempt to impose your thoughts and feelings onto others. If you *give in* (surrender and compromise your position) you usually aim to keep the peace and reduce the conflict. You appear to agree with others even though inside you might disagree. You have a desire to save the situation/relationship even it hurts you. If you *attack* (fight) you tend to impose yourself upon others and their ideas, using condemnation and put-down to discredit them. You have strong emotions and will tell people how you feel about things. Finally, if you *collaborate* (negotiate) you give each party a chance to explain their opinion/position, recognising that everyone has a right to feel the way they do, and you accept differences of opinion. You aim to utilise the strengths of each position and achieve a win-win result. Obviously, the last method is the most productive and should be aimed for whenever possible. The result may not always be exactly what is wanted but if people remain open and willing to learn, almost every conflict situation can be resolved without unnecessary pain and hurt.

Motivating

Motivation is the key to learning. Inspiring individuals to want to learn to perform better is one of the most significant factors in the success of the staff development process. Motivating individuals means creating an environment in which individuals feel they can satisfy their goals. Understanding motivation means understanding the link between goals, energy and reward. 'In an ideal world we would select those individuals whose goals were the same as those of the organisation. We would select those individuals with the energy to pursue these goals persistently, over long periods of time. Finally we would design a reward system which allowed individuals to achieve their goals while at the same time contribute to the goals of the organisation' (Hunt 1986). This obviously does not always occur in practice. First, individuals are often unsure of their goals. Even if there is clarity they can vary widely over time. The goals of individuals are rarely the same as those of the organisation, as the goals for both can change unpredictably. Second, energy levels within individuals vary with length of employment, experience in employment, and personal factors and situations. Third, the official reward systems, that is, money, promotion and free time, is linked to the average individual and has little or no direct effect on motivation.

A number of theories about motivation have been developed (Steers & Porter, 1989). They are discussed briefly here to provide insight into the way people react and therefore to increase awareness for the role.

Drive-reduction theories (1920s)

Individuals are motivated to do things to restore the balance in their environment. When applied to staff development this theory proposes that individuals will feel unbalanced if they don't know something, or if their environment is unbalanced and will be motivated to learn to restore the balance. It is difficult to explain all behaviour in these terms, but it has some useful application. The request for staff development may arise from an experience where knowledge or expertise was lacking and the individual felt uncomfortable, or, according to this theory, unbalanced.

Maslow's theory of hierarchy of needs (1940s)

Maslow highlights social motivators which lack a physiological cause, placing them in a five level hierarchy and arguing that needs at level 1 must be met before level 2, and so on. The levels are:

1 Basic physiological
2 Safety
3 Belongingness (social affiliation)
4 Esteem (appraising, value)
5 Self actualisation (full potential).

Maslow's theory has been enormously influential (Handy 1981), but empirically it is not well established. The five independent levels have been questioned, as has been the hierarchy. In contrast Alderfer (1969 in Handy 1981) uses a classification of three levels of need, existence, relatedness, and growth in order from simple to complex. The implication of order, as in either of these two theories, involves the realisation that an individual cannot be expected to learn beyond their level of development.

Herzberg's theory of job enrichment

Herzberg's theory states that satisfaction is dependent on two independent factors; first, motivators and second, dissatisfiers. Motivators relate to intrinsic factors such as a sense of achievement, recognition, sense of responsibility, and appreciation. Dissatisfiers result from an absence of sufficient hygiene factors, (basic conditions) such as job salary, security, status and working conditions. These two factors are not dependent; for example, providing sufficient hygiene factors may prevent dissatisfaction but it won't necessarily create satisfaction. Applied to staff development this means that increasing opportunities for learning through staff development may satisfy staff, but will not necessarily improve their performance or motivate them to continue to learn.

McClelland's theory of achievement motivation (1960s)

Achievement motivation has two components—the hope for success and the fear of failure. McClelland found close correlation between groups with high levels of achievement motivation and economic growth. He proposed that characteristics of high achievement motivated people can be recognised, these being nonconformity, time consciousness, briskness, and mobility. Achievement motivation can be viewed as the drive for success. In staff development this means people who wish to be successful are more likely to be motivated to learn, or to improve their performance.

Process theories of motivation

Theorists turned to processes to understand motivation in the 1970s. For example, Vroom's expectancy theory recognises three phases of motivation. First, effort is linked to performance: *If I attend this workshop my performance will improve.* Second, performance is linked to outcomes: *If my performance improves I will get recognition.* Third, the outcomes is evaluated and considered worthwhile: *Recognition means more responsibility and possibly promotion.* If the chain breaks down then motivation lessens and learning is unlikely. If applied to staff development, it means that individuals need to see learning as meaningful for them and to be able to identify a purposeful outcome.

None of the theories has been able to explain all situations. As a result a pragmatic approach is often adopted to identify what satisfies and dissatisfies individuals, where individuals rate these factors in order of importance. The assumption is made that if job satisfaction is increased, improved motivation and performance will follow. This presumed link between job satisfaction and motivation is tenuous at best. Locke's work (1979 in Handy 1981) showed salary to be the most effective motivator, goal setting second, job satisfaction third and participation in decision making fourth. As far as staff development is concerned, what becomes evident is the importance of getting to know individuals in order to determine their motivators and to not make assumptions or generalisations based upon presumed behaviour or past experience. The task for the individual in a staff development role is to:

- Identify the goals of individuals and link the task/event to their goals.
- Link the goals to the resources that are necessary and the effort that is required to motivate, inspire, and uplift individuals to accept what has to be done to achieve their goals.

- Design a reward system that is meaningful, to include such factors as friendship, fellowship, identification, recognition, power, autonomy, creativity, or growth.

Then the process of staff development becomes linked to the outcomes of learning, or improved performance.

Self-management

The multiple demands of a staff development role call for considerable self-management ability. This includes management of your personal behaviour as well as management of the work load and activities. Anyone who wants to improve the way they work must manage from the inside out, that is, manage the inner (self) and then outer (other) environment. (Pedlar, Boydell 1985) recognises three states in self-management and describes them as:

- surviving; keeping going in adversity
- maintaining; getting ready for development; being prepared for growth and change
- developing; bring out potential, actual growth and advancement.

He argues there are four personal traits which we need to maintain and develop. He describes them as health (a sound mind and body), skills (mental, technical, social, artistic), action (getting things done in the world) and identity (knowing who you are, accepting yourself while knowing who you want to be). According to Handy (1981), in an age of ever rapid change and redundant skills and knowledge, the individual must take responsibility for his/her own learning and future. This self development implies that the individual will have:

- a clear idea of ultimate priorities and directions
- self knowledge which exposes themself to a range of opportunities and experiences, thereby exploring rather than protecting the self concept
- a willingness to regard the present as an investment in the future, to remain committed to growth and to seek out continual replenishment.

Management of your personal behaviour (inner self) requires a number of competencies (Woodcock, Francis 1982). The competencies are identified as:

- sound personal values
- clear personal objectives
- a commitment to personal growth
- effective problem solving techniques
- capacity to be creative and innovative
- capacity to influence others
- insight into work behaviour
- ability to work with others
- awareness of sources of stress

- realistic expectations of your self
- the ability to take time out to re-energise
- strategies for personal release, debriefing, and resolution.

Management of your work behaviour requires the development of effective work practices. This is often referred to as 'time management'. You can not actually manage time but you can manage how you use time. Referring to the learning as 'time management' (external) tends to take the awareness away from where it is really needed, which is to learn better work practices and behaviour (internal). The first step in learning to manage your time better is to identify your time wasters, those activities and events that waste your time. Time wasters can be classified as external and internal time wasters.

External time wasters	Internal time wasters
Meetings	Disorganisation
Telephone calls	Procrastination
Visitors	Not saying no
Paper work	Lack of delegation
Distractions	Lack of goals
Routine menial tasks	Not listening
Poor communication	Over commitment
Incomplete information	Unrealistic time frames
Problem people	Lack of planning

Not dealing with time wasters can result in poor work practices. There are many common poor work practices which everyone can relate to. Rate yourself on this list.

Characteristics of poor work practices

- always rushing
- chronic vacillation between unpleasant tasks
- chronic fatigue or listlessness
- constantly missing deadlines
- insufficient time for personal relationships
- sense of being overwhelmed
- feeling you are always doing what you do not want to do
- no end in sight
- forgetfulness

The most difficult task in learning to manage your work behaviour effectively involves self reflection. When did you last examine the way you work? Self reflection can be implemented in a systematic, logical way. The following self-management plan is most effective.

Self-management plan

- Compile a log of all your activities for at least one week, listing everything you do.
- Try to identify habits and patterns (eating at the same time, feeling lethargic in the afternoon, working effectively in the early morning).
- Analyse your log and group activities into primary (very important), secondary (fairly important) and tertiary activities (not important).
- Develop a plan that sets your goals for one year (long term), one month (midterm) and one week (short term).
- Set priorities: top drawer items (essential, must be done), middle drawer (can be put off for a while but still important) and bottom drawer (easily put off without harm).
- Match your goals to your priorities. Sometimes this requires accepting that someone else's priority is more important than yours.
- Identify any activities that do not relate to your goals and priorities and get rid of them (delegate, modify, rearrange).
- Adopt behaviours that will allow you to make the most out of the time that is available; learn to say no; banish bottom drawer items; build in time for interruptions, unforeseen problems and unscheduled events; set aside time for personal reflection and space; plan periods of time with no interruptions to work on jobs that require focus; reward achievement; be prepared to review and adjust.

Communicating

Effective communication both verbal—spoken and written, and nonverbal, is a key skill in staff development. Effective communication centres on the concept of transmission of messages between a sender and receiver so that *the message that is received is identical to the one that is sent.* Messages, therefore, need to be sent at the right time, to the right people, and in the right form. Communication is ineffective if the message is too early, too late; sent to too many or too few or to the wrong people; or if its meaning is not clearly understood. Robbins (1986) identifies four functions of communication, all of which have application to the staff development process. They are control, motivation, emotional expression, and information.

There are many barriers to effective communication. What people say can be different from what they mean to say and still different from what the receiver hears or interprets. Apart from actual distortions of words or sounds, common barriers to effective communication can be identified as:

- filtering: the sender manipulates information so that it is seen more favourably by the receiver
- selective perception: the receiver hears and selects out what they want to, partly based upon expectation and/or experience
- emotions: how the receiver feels at the time will influence how the communication is received

- context of relationship: messages are received and interpreted against a background relationship that already exists between the parties com‑municating
- language: words mean different things to different people, and they are emotionally charged, for example, duties, appraise, expectation.

If these are common barriers to effective communication, what skills are necessary to overcome them?

Skills for effective communication

Strong self concept: believe what you communicate is important and valued by the receivers.

Active listening: empathise with and interpret the feelings of the sender.

Clarity of expression: simplify the language; speak and write clearly.

Cope with emotion: channel and contain anger; use reason to control feeling.

Self disclosure: admit own strengths and the need for learning.

Use feedback: check understanding by questioning.

Use nonverbal cues: nonverbal cues can reinforce the verbal messages.

Effective communicators in an organisation tend to be higher in self esteem, more open to change, more influential, more interesting and placed more centrally to the communication network within the organisation. Effective communicators keep messages simple, and avoid overloading the information-processing capacity of the audience. Finally, effective communication also depends on the credibility, persuasion, apparent expertise, and speed and clarity of speech of the communicator.

Written communication in an organisation comes in many forms but regardless of the form, the principles for effective written communication remain the same:

Principles of effective written communication

- The purpose is clearly identified early in the document, preferably the first paragraph.
- The facts are correct.
- The content is concise, logical and meaningful.
- The language is appropriate for the audience.
- The text is technically correct; spelling, grammar, syntax.
- The sender and receiver are clearly identified.
- The required action or response is clearly identified.
- The presentation is simple and clear

Written communication is an essential part of any organisation, but it should be used only where it is necessary and/or the most appropriate means at the time. It should not be used to avoid personal contact, because the sender is lazy and can't be bothered getting around to the receivers, as a means of power and authority, or to avoid accountability and/or explanation.

Technical skills

Technical skills for the staff development role are more readily learnt than interpersonal skills because they can be taught using models and plans. Interpersonal skills however require more complex learning and a change to longstanding behaviour. General technical skills in this sense include planning, organising, delegating, problem solving and decision making, and leadership. Technical skills may also be specific to a position; for example, budgeting, program design and evaluation. Those skills that are most readily applied are delegating, problem solving and decision making, and leadership.

Delegating

Delegating, considered as both a technical and human skill, links authority to accountability. It is the interpersonal component of delegating that often causes problems in organisations. The poorest delegaters will usually freely admit that this is one of their worst skills, yet they continue to hold on to tasks that they know should be delegated. Few people learn how to delegate as part of any aspect of formal education, although the skills required can be taught and developed. The sheer weight of accountability eventually forces individuals to learn to delegate to others. Some individuals never learn and continue throughout their entire career doing everything themselves. They overload themselves and work ineffectively, at the same time inhibiting the growth and potential effectiveness of others with whom they work.

Delegating involves the process of allocating appropriate types of decisions to appropriate people and requires structures and processes to ensure effectiveness. Delegation means the authority has been transferred to someone else. There is some debate as to where the final responsibility lies, when delegation occurs. Some organisations believe the more senior position retains ultimate responsibility, while others believe the responsibility goes with the delegation. It is essential that the responsibility and authority is clearly spelt out at every stage, including the responsibility for decision making. This is crucial in health care organisations where many decisions involve life-and death situations.

Ineffective delegation is characterised by:

- withholding of information
- insufficient information
- unclear or incomplete messages
- insufficient resources to carry out the action
- ineffective or lack of strategies
- unrealistic and unclear outcomes
- interfering
- overruling actions and/or decisions
- censure for unacceptable results

- lack of opportunities for growth.

Effective delegating requires the following skills and attitudes:

- commitment to the process and outcome of delegation
- careful analysis of each situation where delegation is contemplated
- communication of all relevant information
- clear instructions/guidelines for the process and outcome
- clearly defined outcomes
- demonstrated trust in the individual to whom you have delegated
- delegation of the action, accountability and responsibility.

Delegation and being able to receive delegation are essential skills in staff development and part of total commitment to learning and growth and characterises the staff development process. Incomplete delegation, that is, activities but not responsibility, inhibits the real performance of others and provides confusing messages about perceived and actual performance expectations.

Problem solving and decision making

Problem solving requires the making of a decision and so the two behaviours are considered together. Problem solving, the first part of the process and decision making, the second part, take a number of stages. They are:

- identifying potential problems (*problem solving*)
- articulating and diagnosing actual problems
- evaluating and/or generating alternative solution
- choosing the best solution for the situation (*decision making*)
- implementing the chosen solution
- evaluating the result.

This methodical and rational process is often ignored in favour of a hurried approach that involves collecting information, searching through experience for alternatives, and making a decision and acting. This action may solve the immediate problem but as it is not based on thorough analysis, it is unlikely to be a long term solution.

In some organisations, managing is seen to be all about solving problems. Merely solving problems is not, however, the key to successful performance. Decisions must also be made. Problems can also be opportunities, arising from a single event or insight into a situation. For both problems and opportunities, information will be collected until there is enough to make a decision. What is enough is clearly related to the individual's willingness to take risks, and to feel confident with the judgement that has been made. The ability to collect information (the process of solving the problem) and the level of information people feel they need before they can make a decision, varies from person to person. Some people, given to procrastination, persist in collecting information until the opportunity has come and gone and a new problem has arisen. Making no decision at all is not necessarily procrastination; many problems resolve themselves. Procrastination is deferring action when action is needed, when a decision needs to be made. The mental process of making a decision has interested researchers for some time, but few useful decision making models have been found to be particularly useful. The way a decision is made is dependent upon the interpersonal characteristics and behaviour patterns of each individual.

The following guidelines look at how to achieve each stage of a problem solving and decision making process in more detail:

Effective problem solving and decision making

Problem solving

Identify potential problems: sometimes referred to as a trouble shooter role	*look for deviations from expectations* *listen to the staff* *monitor the market place* *back your judgement and your intuition* *remain in touch with everyday activities.*
Articulate and diagnose actual problems:	*accept the evidence* *take action, avoid procrastination* *speak up early and clearly* *look for reasons and sources of information to explain and understand* *anticipate potential events or situations.*
Evaluate and/or generate alternatives:	*look for experience* *be creative and innovative* *evaluate all the options;* *justify the choice with evidence* *avoid re-inventing the wheel.*

Decision making

Choose the best solution:	*consider if a problem that has re-occurred* *consider if a new problem with no past experience* *be flexible and realistic* *be prepared to learn from mistakes* *communicate clearly, openly, and fully.*
Implement the solution:	*involve all relevant parties* *plan the action* *be decisive but realistic* *maintain a formal, written record* *explain the process and outcomes.*
Evaluate the result:	*collect evidence of outcomes* *obtain comments from individuals* *compare the initial situation against the result* *look for clear evidence.*

Because of the emphasis on people within the staff development role, it is not uncommon to find that a perceived problem situation is actually caused by a *problem person*. Within any organisation there are individuals who appear to have all the problems. Everyone else seems to spend a lot of time helping the person with the problem rather than getting on with their own work. We all like to help when we can and can become embroiled in the problem person's (self created) problems without realising the effect that they are having on us and/or the group. The problem person needs to be identified and does need assistance. You need to look at whether the person has an agenda of *trying to fail* as opposed to *working at succeeding*. If attempts to assist the person continue to be unsuccessful and you still feel you are just waiting for a problem to happen with this person, it could be that the person consciously or unconsciously has no intention of being assisted and wants to stay with their current behaviour.

People with problems can have a damaging effect on organisations and have the potential to counteract growth and development with a group. Problem people do not necessarily present as nasty people nor display aggressive behaviour. They may have adopted a dependent behaviour to avoid dealing with an inability to cope or just feel unable to make decisions or to be accountable. Recognising problem people can break a cycle of unproductive behaviour and turn the organisation around to a more positive approach. In many cases the person will not be aware of their behaviour so that action will be necessary. Frequently, the behaviour of a problem person arises from a lack of confidence, fear of failure and severe self criticism. If it is manipulative behaviour on their part, then it will be necessary to break the pattern. These guidelines should assist you to effectively deal with a problem person:

- Identify the person and their behaviour patterns.
- Identify the responses of others to this person.
- Identify any pattern to situations where problems seem to arise.
- Confirm your assessment with others.
- Arrange for their performance to be formally assessed (performance appraisal).
- Interview the problem person as part of the appraisal and outline the behaviour that is of concern. Make sure you can provide actual examples.
- Use the interview as an opportunity to find out about the person's goals, interests, and job satisfaction.
- Invite the person to identify how the behaviour can be changed. Aim to achieve consensus of opinion but if necessary, be assertive.
- Set goals for changing behaviour giving consideration to ways to mobilise the person's ability and interest.
- Establish a time frame for review.

Leadership

Leadership can be described as the ability to influence a group toward the achievement of goals. This influence may be over people's attitudes, behaviours, or opinions. There is no all-embracing leadership theory; instead there are many theories that compete and complement each other. Leadership theories can be clustered into four major categories.

1 Trait theories: the identification of behaviour traits that leaders possess
2 Behavioural theories: the identification of specific behaviours that identify leaders
3 Situational or contingency theories: the identification of the relationship between style and situation
4 Applied theories: the inter-relationship between traits, behaviours of the person leading, situations, and the characteristics of those who are to be led.

Although the study of leadership theories is not particularly useful here, there are ingredients for leadership behaviour that are more useful. They are:

- the power and influence of the leader (rather than the authority)
- the understanding of people, especially the ability to motivate people to get the desired response
- the ability to inspire support, loyalty and effort over and above that needed to meet individual need
- the ability to develop a climate for leadership
- the behaviour style of the leader.

In the staff development role, leadership mostly relates to the ability to influence learning and performance. Being a leader also involves setting an example for behaviour and this aspect of leadership is also important in the staff development role. When a person makes a suggestion, gives an order, or makes a decision to other members of a group, that person is exercising leadership. This leadership will be accepted if there is some justification for the claim, based upon knowledge, experience, appointment or position, or personal qualities.

The staff development role provides many opportunities where leadership can be exercised. It is important to note the distinction between leadership and authority. A position not a person is invested with authority. Staff may reject a person's leadership, yet still follow orders on the basis of their authority. On the other hand, a person may be perceived to be a leader (an informal position) but not have authority (formal position) within an organisation. This latter situation may cause difficulty if the support is for the 'informal' leader.

To demonstrate leadership behaviour, you need to have the following characteristics. You need to be:

- energetic
- a high achiever
- goal-directed
- organised
- able to work alone

- confident
- self-reflective
- assertive.

It has been clearly established that the staff development role is important to the growth of the organisation. Therefore, the individual in a staff development role is very likely to assume a leadership role, either within individual activities and situations, or within the organisation in general.

Conceptual skills

The capacity to *see the big picture*, to see the whole situation, is not widely distributed. It is this ability to conceptualise that facilitates the linking together of all the stages of the staff development process. It is, therefore, a crucial skill for the staff development role. The behavioural outcomes of the ability to conceptualise can be identified as the ability to:

- articulate corporate staff development values and beliefs
- design a corporate staff development structure
- integrate staff development systems and processes to avoid unnecessary competition
- select staff development techniques
- design integrated programs
- give and receive feedback
- relate evaluation to objectives
- learn from every situation.

Conceptual skills are difficult to teach as they involve the capacity to process information broadly and specifically. The processes that are involved are partly genetic, partly a product of upbringing and environment, and partly learned as a product of education and/or experience. Courses in strategic planning, for example, attempt to develop conceptual skills but have questionable success. Models and checklists force participants to investigate parts of the problem, but do little to help people to *see the big picture*.

Some of the most interesting research has arisen from work done in the area of whole-brain learning, where individuals are encouraged to develop the ability to use both right and left brain hemisphere function (Rose 1985). The ability to be able to see the big picture is influenced by the ability to use both hemispheres of the brain. Western society traditionally encourages left-hemisphere function, as represented in the use of analytical, logical, mathematical, sequential thinking. This tends to discard the significance of right-hemisphere function, as represented in the use of imagination, pictures, shapes, symbols, creativity and spatial thinking. Conceptual skills depend on the ability to use the whole brain for analysis and performance. Research (Gardner 1993) has shown that the right brain or hemisphere, referred to as the creative brain, processes information 40-400 times faster than the left hemisphere of the brain, the analytical side of the brain. Research (Gardner 1993) has also shown that memory takes place with left and right hemisphere communication, the linking of words and pictures. Accelerated learning, which is an application of whole-brain learning, is a method of tapping into the preferred learning style of as many people as possible, some of the time (see Ch. 3).

One application of whole-brain learning of particular value in the development of conceptual skills is referred to as *mind mapping* (sometimes referred to as mind charting and mind scapes). Mind mapping is a way of recording information effectively so that both left and right hemispheres of the brain are operating; that is, linking words to pictures. Mind mapping is the practice of recording, analysing and acting on information through the use of pictures, symbols, key words, and colours, that are personal to the user. A picture or words and symbols is created to form an image that represents a situation, plan, event or learning.

This method has application for staff development. It can be used to develop a writing plan, teaching plan, or strategic plan, or to work through a problem to identify the best solution. It can also be used to develop a study plan, in the preparation of a speech or meeting, in report writing, and in program design. It is an effective way to gather information, analyse options and develop an action plan.

The application of whole brain behaviour can be seen in the following examples, all of which have been achieved in various employment settings. In each case, the approach that was taken aimed to address the big picture.

Example 1: The development of an organisation-wide staff development plan that integrates individual, departmental, organisation and client needs to a common objective. There was a requirement to look at the whole organisation without losing sight of individuals, departments, or clients. It was necessary to look at the whole picture before individual areas could be considered.

Example 2: The design of an education program for a department with multiple streams for different staff categories/classifications but including common components, such as an introduction to the organisation, goals and objectives, and common outcomes in terms of performance expectations. In this case, individual staff groups were considered individually, but the overall program linked them together as part of the whole organisation.

Example 3: An organisation-wide performance appraisal strategy and documentation that can be used for every staff member, regardless of position, which appraises performance on common standards, at appropriate levels, and includes individualised goal setting and performance planning. In this case the issue performance appraisal was considered from an organisation-wide point of view; that is, the big picture was considered.

The possession of conceptual skills is more significant in the staff development role than either specific human or technical skills. The appointment of a *big picture person* to an organisation in a staff development role is an enormous advantage.

Recommended formal qualifications and experience

It is difficult to identify specific formal qualifications for the staff development role. There are, however, a number of areas in which qualifications and experience are recommended. Because a considerable part of the staff development process involves personnel type functions, qualifications and experience in human resource management would be considered relevant, but not necessarily essential.

Some qualifications and experience can be recommended for the staff development role in a health care organisation. This list may be useful in defining a job description and/or the selection of personnel:

Formal qualifications in a health related discipline
This should provide a foundation for understanding health care services, the client population, the employee characteristics, and ensure a level of knowledge.

Considerable practical experience in a health care discipline
This facilitates an understanding of work practices, a realistic understanding of service demand and delivery, client needs and actual staff performance.

Formal qualifications in education
As staff development involves growth and development and the facilitation of learning, this is an essential area. Experience in a range of education roles would be an advantage.

Management qualifications and experience, particularly human service management
The role has a significant management component and therefore knowledge of management processes and practices would be an advantage. Experience in a senior management position is not necessarily as useful.

Qualifications in a behavioural discipline (psychology, sociology, behavioural science)
Staff development focuses on interaction with people and qualifications and experience in this area would enhance performance in the role.

Personal attributes
I consider the following six attributes are essential for a role in staff development:

Essential attributes

- effective communicator
- high level of self-management
- ability to conceptualise—a big picture person
- ability to be creative and innovative
- high level of organisation and planning
- ability to work alone with minimum supervision, but with regard for others.

With an understanding of the staff development role and essential behaviours for the role, it is possible for an organisation to understand how to get the most from the staff development role. Performance in the staff development role will be maximised with:

- clearly defined role and responsibilities
- clear and realistic expectations for performance
- adequate human, material and financial resources
- autonomy and independence within agreed parameters
- challenge and opportunity
- recognition and status within the organisation.

Chapter summary

The staff development role will vary between organisations and between departments within organisations, according to the organisation's structure and management model/strategy. It is difficult to identify specific formal qualifications for the role, but there are certainly personal qualities, skills and experiences that will enhance performance in the role. This chapter has discussed personal qualities for effective performance, likening them to those qualities identified for effective management of human resources. Essential behaviours were discussed in terms of three components of the role: a relating role, an informational role and a decision role. Skills for the role were discussed in three groups: human skills, technical skills and conceptual skills. Finally, recommended qualifications and experience for a role in staff development were identified. With consideration given to all these factors, an organisation should be able obtain the most benefit from the staff development role.

REFERENCES

Donovan F, Jackson A 1991 Managing human service organisations. Prentice Hall, Sydney

Gardner H 1993 Frames of mind. Paladin, New York

Handy C B 1981 Understanding organisations. Penguin, London

Hunt J W 1986 Managing peoples at work: a manager's guide to behaviour in organisations. McGraw-Hill, London

Pedler M, Boydell P 1985 Managing yourself. Fontana, USA

Robbins A 1986 Unlimited power. Simon & Schuster

Rose C 1985 Frames of mind. Accelerated Learning Systems, London

Steers R M, Porter L W , 1989 Motivation and work behaviour. McGraw-Hill, Sydney

Woodcock M, Francis D 1982 The unblocked manager. Gower, London

9

Practical examples and resources

Key questions

- What types of questions can be included in a needs assessment questionnaire?
- What is a teaching plan?
- What does a performance appraisal evaluation form look like?
- How could I structure a short course?
- How can I organise a speech?

Content summary

Introduction

Questions for a needs assessment questionnaire

Relaxation exercise for the release of occupational or personal stress

Writing objectives

Developing a teaching plan

Evaluation

Performance appraisal

Didactic presentation

Meeting planning and evaluation

Interactive workshop

Short courses
   Short course for women
   Short course for managers

Preparing for a presentation
   Presentation evaluation

Resources

Introduction

Many examples have been included throughout the book, as part of the discussion. There have been, however, some topics where it has not been practical to include an example within the chapter. This chapter brings together further examples that may be useful for the reader as they implement a role in staff development. In some situations, the examples that are given may also provide guidelines for further development. In almost all cases, the examples are from my own work, presented here because they have been found to be effective. Finally, there is a list of further resources, including books, journals, and samples of music that have been used an aid to learning.

Questions for a needs assessment questionnaire

Needs assessment has been described as a most significant component of the staff development process. The instrument that has been discussed in detail, the questionnaire, is most common and provides a mechanism to obtain a large quantity of general data as well as some specific data. Figure 9.1 is an example of a question that aims to measure *personal education needs*. Figure 9.2 is an example of a question that aims to measure *perceptions of management*. Figure 9.3 is an example of an *open question*, that aims to provide an opportunity for the respondent to make comments on any other topic of their choice. These examples were all taken from *a needs assessment survey instrument* used in an organisation-wide staff development research project.

Q8 PERSONAL EDUCATION

How important is it for you personally to increase your understanding of these topics? Please choose ONE number for EACH topic.

VERY IMPORTANT - VI	1
MODERATELY IMPORTANT - MI	2
LITTLE IMPORTANCE - LI	3
NOT IMPORTANT - NI	4

	VI	MI	LI	NI
Problem solving skills	1	2	3	4
Assertiveness	1	2	3	4
Community resources for clilents	1	2	3	4
Effective communications	1	2	3	4
Managing stress at work	1	2	3	4
Setting goals	1	2	3	4
Establishing priorities	1	2	3	4
Legal issues	1	2	3	4
Ethical issues in care	1	2	3	4
Car maintenance	1	2	3	4
Conflict resolution	1	2	3	4
Career planning	1	2	3	4
Planning for retirement	1	2	3	4
Study skills	1	2	3	4

Fig. 9.1 Example of a question that aims to measure personal education needs

Q32 Think about your immediate leader or manager in your current job. Please circle ONE response for each statement.

STRONG AGREEMENT - SA	1
MODERATE AGREEMENT - MA	2
AGREEMENT - A	3
DISAGREEMENT - D	4
MODERATE DISAGREEMENT - MD	5
STRONG DISAGREEMENT - SD	6

	SA	MA	A	D	MD	SD
I am told precisely what is expected of me in my job	1	2	3	4	5	6
There are clear criteria against which my performance can be measured	1	2	3	4	5	6
I get sufficient feedback on how well I do my job	1	2	3	4	5	6
My leader is consistent in their approach	1	2	3	4	5	6
Problems are dealt with in a calm, constructive way	1	2	3	4	5	6
I have freedom to do my job as I like to	1	2	3	4	5	6
I feel I have authority over people I am responsible for	1	2	3	4	5	6
Poor performance is not tolerated	1	2	3	4	5	6
I have authority to act upon work delegated to me	1	2	3	4	5	6
I am consulted before decisions are made	1	2	3	4	5	6

Fig. 9.2 Example of a question that aims to measure perceptions of management

Question

Is there anything at all that you would like to comment on in relation to your current job? Please write your comments in this space provided. Your honest comments would be appreciated.

Fig. 9.3 Example of an open question

Relaxation exercise for the release of occupational or personal stress

Occupational stress is one of three common themes of need identified in health care organisations (see Ch. 2). There are as many ways to handle occupational stress as there are sources of occupational stress. As an individual, you may need to look to change your behaviour, adopt a more realistic approach to your performance, or develop a technique to reduce your reaction to the symptoms of stress. In the staff development role, you may need to present a session on ways to manage symptoms of stress.

A simple yet effective technique to present is a *spot meditation* exercise (Fig. 9.4). This exercise can be used at home, sitting in the car at the end or beginning of the work day, or sitting at your desk. I have developed this exercise and used it for my own personal use and within many workshops. It is best accompanied in the early stages by some quiet relaxing music to help to eliminate external noise and/or distraction, but music is not necessary. It can be completed in less than ten minutes, with an effective result. If you are using this exercise with a group, the following guidelines will help:

*   Introduce the exercise as part of the management of symptoms of stress.
*   If possible, dim the lights and prevent any interruptions.
*   Ask people to find a relaxed position, either sitting or lying down.
*   Commence playing the music and let it play quietly for about 30 seconds.
*   Begin to speak slowly and with an even pitch to your voice.
*   Talk the people through the exercise.

Allow people to remain in their relaxed position for a few minutes at the completion of the exercise, before moving onto the next activity.

Writing objectives

Any learning activity requires objectives. Objectives describe the outcome that is required at the completion of the activity; the change in behaviour or attitude that is expected, or the knowledge that will result. An objective must:

*   describe the final result
*   be specific and precise
*   describe a change that is measurable and observable.
    The following terms are commonly used when writing an objective.

Common terms for objectives			
classify	determine	evaluate	integrate
construct	differentiate	explain	list
define	discuss	specify	name
describe	distinguish	identify	practise
designate	establish	indicate	state

SPOT MEDITATION
For immediate relief of stress symptoms

Step 1: **Recognise your need and take action**

Stop what you are doing and sit or stand still, scan your body posture and identify tightness and tension

Become aware of your breathing and consciously slow it down

Take five deep slow breaths

Release the tightness and tension with each breath

Notice how your body has become softer.

Step 2: **Complete a body scan**

Divide the body into seven parts and examine each part as you move through your body

Feel the tension; breath through the tension–release the tension.

1   scalp and forehead
2   face and lower part of the head
3   neck, throat, shoulders
4   chest, arms and hands
5   back and buttocks
6   diaphragm, solar plexus and gut
7   hips, legs and feet

Step 3: **Focus meditation**

Complete the release of tightness and tension

Focus on some part of your body–wherever your mind settles

Focus on your breathing as it moves in and out of your body, for five full breaths

Focus only on your breathing

Notice how completely relaxed you have become and recognise how that feels

Remain in this relaxed state for as long as you need to.

Step 4: **Stretch, energise and face the world**

Open your eyes and stretch the whole body

Resume your activity

Fig. 9.4 Spot meditation exercise

When writing objectives it is useful to begin with this statement . At *the end of this session, the learner will be able to*..... The following examples of objectives are provided.

Learning objectives

Learning: Clinical learning session on medication administration

Objectives: List all ten basic rules of medication administration;
Describe the process for checking the identity of the patient before administering medications;
Explain the most common errors made when administering medications.

Learning: The role of the health professional

Objectives: Discuss the concept of professionalism;
Debate current ethical and legal issues within your area of practice;
Identify effective leadership behaviour;
Apply techniques which identify and resolve conflict between health professionals.

Developing a teaching plan

There are many different things to think about when preparing to present an educational session. Your planning should begin with the development of a teaching plan. This simple teaching plan shows a basic approach but it is useful as a beginning, and can be elaborated upon with experience.

Teaching plan

Title: State the title of the session. This assists to keep you to the topic.

Target group: help to identify if you know your group well.

Learning needs: Determine what it is you want the learners to gain from this session. Consider their needs as well as your own.

Objectives: Write the learning objectives.

Content: Outline the content of the session using broad headings and then specific details.

Methods: Determine the medhod(s) you will use, the equipment you will need; the resources required. Pay attention to detail.

Schedule: Determine the time frame, including breaks and activities.

Evaluation: Determine the method of evaluation you intend to use and prepare any necessary materials.

Evaluation

There are many different ways to evaluate a learning session. The form that is presented here provides some useful information (Fig. 9.5).

Education Evaluation

Please indicate your response to the following statements by circling ONE of the numbers in the scale below.

1 The information was easy to follow and understand
Strongly agree   1   2   3   4   Strongly disagree

2 The method of presentation was effective
Strongly agree   1   2   3   4   Strongly disagree

3 The areas of the topic that I wanted to know about were covered
Strongly agree   1   2   3   4   Strongly disagree

4 The information provided was relevant to the topic
Strongly agree   1   2   3   4   Strongly disagree

5 Indicate the most useful topics that were covered
....

6 Indicate what else you would have liked covered
....

7 How could this session be improved?
....

Fig. 9.5 Evaluation form

Performance appraisal

Many different performance appraisal forms are in use in health care organisations. The example that is presented here was developed for use by all staff within a domiciliary health care organisation (Fig. 9.6). Key performance areas are classified into three performance standards; pro–fessionalism, communication and management. Components of behaviour within each standard are developed and defined. The individual's performance is appraised (assessed) by two people, one being the individual themself and the other, the most appropriate for this person's position. In many cases, more than one person will assess and all information is taken into account. Performance is evaluated on a scale of 1-5 and each level is explained. Finally, learning needs are identified and goals for future development are established. The advantages of an organisation-wide form include:

• key standards for the organisation are established and evaluated consistently
• appraisal is uniform and measures the same standards across the organisation
• staff become familiar with the form and comfortable with its use
• overall organisation performance can be evaluated, that is, against the key standards.

PERFORMANCE APPRAISAL

NAME: ....

CURRENT POSITION: ....

DATE: ....

DATE OF LAST REVIEW: ....

This document is designed by all staff within the Association. It should function as a guide for communication between appraiser and appraisee, to recognise performance and to promote further growth and development.

Steps for use

1   Decide the expected level of performance for the position

2   The appraisee and the appraiser should each complete a form

3   Both documents then form the basis of discussion

4   One form remains in the staff file

5   One form remains with the staff member for future reference.

On the following page is a list of words that describe behaviour in the work environment. They have been grouped according to performance standards of

PROFESSIONALISM   COMMUNICATION   MANAGEMENT

Each word has been defined.

You are asked to choose the number that best describes your work performance, for each word.

VERY IMPORTANT: Different positions will have different expectations as represented by the numbers 1-5

Numbers describe performance

5   PERFORMANCE GOES SIGNIFICANTLY BEYOND JOB REQUIREMENTS

4   PERFORMANCE GOES WELL BEYOND JOB REQUIREMENTS

3   PERFORMANCE IS AS EXPECTED FOR THE POSITION

2   PERFORMANCE COULD BE IMPROVED

1   PERFORMANCE IS NOT SATISFACTORY

Fig. 9.6 Performance appraisal

DESCRIPTION OF TERMS

JOB KNOWLEDGE — Familiarity and understanding of the job requirements, received through education or practical experience

HUMAN RELATIONS — Friendliness, enthusiasm, poise and consideration for others and acknowledgement of the importance of the team concept

ATTENDANCE — Ability to be on the job during regular hours of work

STRESS MANAGEMENT — Ability to recognise causes of stress in self and others and implement appropriate strategies to ensure work performance

DEPENDABILITY — Extent to which employee can be counted on to carry out instructions, be on the job on time and fulfil job responsibilities

DECISIVENESS — Ability to make decisions, take action and follow through

MARKETING ABILITY — Presentation of ones self and on behalf of the organisation in the pursuit of satisfactory colleague and client interaction

FLEXIBILITY — Willingness and ability to adjust to changes in job requirements

COMMUNICATION — Ability to converse with colleagues and clients in a problem solving manner, concerning ideas, instructions and plans. (If management, the ability to train others)

CO-OPERATION — Ability and willingness to work in harmony with others toward organisational and individual goals

DELEGATION — Ability to effectively assign work to others

LEADERSHIP — Ability to lead and influence employees in developing and maintaining a high standard of excellence

ORGANISATION — Ability to effectively organise time and effort on work

FORWARD PLANNING — Ability to plan ahead in order to meet changing needs

COMPREHENSION — Ability to understand explanations, master routines and recognise the intentions of others

INITIATIVE — Ability to instigate new initiatives, perform without constant supervision and to be resourceful and self reliant

QUALITY OF WORK — Neatness, accuracy and thoroughness of work with a view to client related quality outcomes

QUANTITY OF WORK — Appropriate need specific work outcomes

COST CONSCIOUSNESS — Ability to use human, financial and physical resources wisely

CREATIVITY — Ability to think in broad perspective, anticipate problems and conceive new ideas and techniques

PERFORMANCE EVALUATION

Appraisee input   **Appraiser input**

STANDARD ONE
(Professionalism))

Appraisee						Appraiser				
1 2 3 4 5	Attendance	1 2 3 4 5
1 2 3 4 5	Job knowledge	1 2 3 4 5
1 2 3 4 5	Dependability	1 2 3 4 5
1 2 3 4 5	Initiative	1 2 3 4 5
1 2 3 4 5	Marketing ability	1 2 3 4 5
1 2 3 4 5	Quality of work	1 2 3 4 5

Comments   *Comments*

— — — — — — — — —   — — — — — — — — —

— — — — — — — — —   — — — — — — — — —

— — — — — — — — —   — — — — — — — — —

STANDARD TWO
(Communication)

Appraisee						Appraiser				
1 2 3 4 5	Human relations	1 2 3 4 5
1 2 3 4 5	Stress management	1 2 3 4 5
1 2 3 4 5	Communication	1 2 3 4 5
1 2 3 4 5	Co-operation	1 2 3 4 5
1 2 3 4 5	Leadership	1 2 3 4 5
1 2 3 4 5	Comprehension	1 2 3 4 5

Comments   *Comments*

— — — — — — — — —   — — — — — — — — —

— — — — — — — — —   — — — — — — — — —

— — — — — — — — —   — — — — — — — — —

STANDARD THREE
(Management)

Appraisee						Appraiser				
1 2 3 4 5	Flexibility	1 2 3 4 5
1 2 3 4 5	Decisiveness	1 2 3 4 5
1 2 3 4 5	Delegation	1 2 3 4 5
1 2 3 4 5	Organisation	1 2 3 4 5
1 2 3 4 5	Forward planning	1 2 3 4 5
1 2 3 4 5	Quantity of work	1 2 3 4 5
1 2 3 4 5	Creativity	1 2 3 4 5
1 2 3 4 5	Cost consciousness	1 2 3 4 5

Comments   *Comments*

— — — — — — — — —   — — — — — — — — —

— — — — — — — — —   — — — — — — — — —

— — — — — — — — —   — — — — — — — — —

FOR THE APPRAISEE

Please underline the words that describe your needs in your work environment that are **not currently being met.**

| CHALLENGE | PRAISE | STABILITY | DIRECTION |
| BASIC BENEFITS | RESPECT | VARIETY | INDEPENDENCE |

Goals for future development of performance

Goal	Strategy	Outcome date

Didactic presentation

The example here is a one-day formal session because of the nature of the topic and the information level of the audience (Fig. 9.7). It was a new topic to the group and so there was less opportunity for interaction and discussion, although some small group work was completed. The organisation wanted the session to be informative and to provide an overview of the topic, rather than an indepth analysis. Further sessions followed after this one, where participants spent time developing their own examples for their area of work. These sessions were much more interactive.

From needs assessment to quality outcomes

This session is designed for people involved in education within the organisation. It aims to provide a beginning understanding, background for future planning and development, guidelines for decision making in the area of needs assessment, and to demonstrate how the data from a needs assessment can be used to achieve quality outcomes in the organisation.

Session 1:	**Needs assessment**
	What is needs assessment?
	What is the purpose of needs assessment to the organisation?
	Classifying needs
	How to design a needs assessment tool
Session 2:	**Processing the data**
	Collecting, sorting and classifying the data
	Identifying priority areas
	Employer/employee relationships in needs assessment
Session 3:	**Program design**
	The process of staff development
	Program design
	Content development
	Learning and teaching principles
	The adult learner
Session 4:	**Evaluation**
	Measuring quality outcomes
	Maximising performance by meeting needs
	Organisational efficiency and staff development
	Future planning

Fig. 9.7 Didactic presentation (lecture)

Meeting planning and evaluation

The meeting is an example of a structgured staff development session. There should be some planning for a good meeting. The following planning guide will assist in preparing for a good meeting (Fig. 9.8).

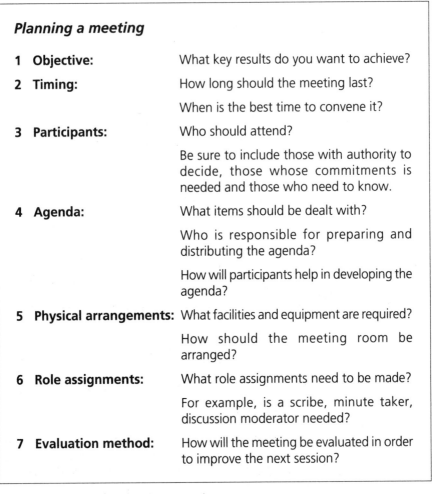

Planning a meeting

1 Objective: What key results do you want to achieve?

2 Timing: How long should the meeting last?

When is the best time to convene it?

3 Participants: Who should attend?

Be sure to include those with authority to decide, those whose commitments is needed and those who need to know.

4 Agenda: What items should be dealt with?

Who is responsible for preparing and distributing the agenda?

How will participants help in developing the agenda?

5 Physical arrangements: What facilities and equipment are required?

How should the meeting room be arranged?

6 Role assignments: What role assignments need to be made?

For example, is a scribe, minute taker, discussion moderator needed?

7 Evaluation method: How will the meeting be evaluated in order to improve the next session?

Fig. 9.8 Worksheet for planning a meeting

Meetings should be evaluated. The benefits of an evaluation will be worthwhile if the following conditions exist:

- The convenor wants to improve future meetings.
- The convenor receives honest input from evaluators.
- Evaluators are candid in their assessment.
- The convenor receives feedback in a positive way.
- The convenor incorporates improvements into future meetings.

The following example is a form that has been used to evaluate a meeting (Fig. 9.9). The questions could be varied to suit any particular situation.

Meeting evaluation form

Based upon your observations and feelings, how would you rate this meeting on the following statements?

1 *To what extent were objectives clearly stated?*

Completely unclear 1   2   3   4   Completely clear

2 *To what extent was the knowledge of the participants utilised?*

Not at all   1   2   3   4   Completely

3 *To what extent was decision making shared by participants?*

Dominated by one 1   2   3   4   Completely shared

4 *To what extent did people trust and level with each other?*

Not at all open   1   2   3   4   Completely open

5 *To what extent were all participants actively involved in the meeting?*

Not at all   1   2   3   4   To a great extent

6 *To what extent did leadership style contribute to meeting effectiveness?*

Not at all   1   2   3   4   To a great extent

Fig. 9.9 Meeting evaluation form

Interactive workshop

The key to the success of an interactive workshop lies in the planning. Once the planning has been completed, the focus can then move to the method and presentation style. The example that is presented here (Fig. 9.10) has several significant features.

- The content of the program is broken down into topics, or chunks of information.
- Each chunk of information has a specific focus..
- The interactive method weaves throughout the program.
- The time is carefully allocated to each chunk of the program.
- A variety of teaching methods are used.

This particular workshop was developed for nurses who were in their first year of nursing since registration. It was part of a *graduate year* program.

Professional issues for the beginning practitioner

9.00-9.15   **Session 1: Introduction and warm up**
Introduction to the topic
Introduction to the methodology
Method: activity and interaction

9.15-10.15   **Session 2: Nursing as a profession**
What is a profession—where does nursing fit?
What is professionalism—identifying behaviours
Challenges for nursing
Barriers to professionalism
Method: working with whole group, involvement and discussion

Posture break—interactive

10.15-10.45   Morning tea

10.45-12.00   **Session 3: Key principles in nursing practice**
1 The meaning of universal precautions in nursing practice
Method: slide presentation
2 Communication—assertive behaviour; male and female interaction
Method: interactive
3 Problem solving—a way of thinking
Method: large group interaction and involvement

12.00-12.30   **Session 4: Today's challenges**
What are the major challenges facing you in your role today?
Method: small groups with feedback

Massage break—interactive

12.30-13.30   Lunch

13.30-14.30   **Session 5: Ethical/moral/legal issues**
Principles in dealing with situations
Interactive hypothetical

14.30-15.15   **Session 6: Presenting yourself**
Your inner self—what you see
Your outer self—what others see
Making everyone a winner—applying for jobs
Method: Interactive

Networking break—interactive

15.15-15.45   Afternoon tea

15.45-16.30   **Session 7: Empowerment and leadership**
The meaning of empowerment
Empowered management
Developing leaders

16.30-17.00   **Session 8: Where to from here?**
Putting ideas into practice
Making a commitment to life long learning
Summary of the day
Method: mixture

Posture/massage/networking

Fig. 9.10 Interactive workshop I

The second example of an interactive workshop demonstrates the use of music to create the learning environment and build the energy within the group, and the use of exercises/activities throughout the program (Fig. 9.11). This workshop was presented as a concurrent session during a conference for health professionals. This example was used by the presenter; the participants were given work books.

Creative stress management—just one more challenge

3.30-5.00pm   *Opening music sequence*

3.00-3.10   **Introduction and icebreakers**
Introduction to me, the session, the method, each other

Communication game

3.10-3.20   **Seize the day—look at your world through different eyes**
Look around the room—take note of the details of the room
Stand on your chairs—now take note of the details of the room, does it look different?
Lie on the floor—now take note of the details of the room, does it look different?
I'm asking you to change your thinking—to look at your world through different eyes, then your behaviour will change
There are some wonderful people in this room—find a partner from these wonderful people (all lying on the floor) and sit together

3.20-3.35   **Pairs activity**
Person A and B
Close your eyes and bring to your mind a recent situation at work when you experienced feelings of stress; recall how you felt; taste, smell, touch how you felt
Describe the situation to your partner
Partner A listen to partner B and then tell the partner what feelings you heard in the story as it was told to you
Reverse the process

3.35-3.45   **Group discussion**
Identify common situations and list on the board
Discuss the common situations
Identify common feelings that were identified and list on the white board

Look for key words

3.45-4.15   **Understanding stress**
Salutogenic model (Aaron Antonovsky)
When you accept that stress is part of living you can learn to manage stress and stay well

Let me help you to feel what I mean.

Analogy: Close your eyes and come on a journey with me.
Let me show you what you can see from the inner side of your eyes.
Dim the lights. Music: Pachobel's Canon.

Raft and waterfall journey

General discussion
You have just experienced the principles that are the foundation of

The salutogenic model: how to manage stress and stay healthy

4.15-4.45   **Stress management models**
Many models of stress management are pathogenic in orientation (disease oriented)—they focus on the identification of risk factors and how to avoid them; focus on what is going wrong when you do not cope.

How can I stop myself going over the waterfall?
How can I identify and avoid the risks in my life so I won't have to be challenged?

This model looks at what is going right: looks for the strengths in behaviour and how people cope in situations.

My journey is full of waterfalls. Look at all those people who are coping—what are they doing that is so successful and what can I do?

Present the model
Based upon a sense of coherence
You will cope when you have a strong sense of coherence (SOC)

Application to work
Identify a situation: rate on the continuum of cohesion

Work through the model:
 can you comprehend it? (sense)
 can you manage it? (resources)
 can you understand it? (make meaning)

When you answer Yes—what is the outcome?
When you answer No—what is the outcome?
What do you need to do to deal better with it (not avoid) next time?

4.30-4.45   **Visualisation**
Revisit the waterfall: Pachobel's Canon

In this moment you have conquered the situation and you have managed the stress. Just one more challenge—that is all it was.

Open your eyes and congratulate the first person you see—give them a hug! Celebrate your success. Trumpets.

Discuss the feelings—open discussion

4.45-5.00   **Recap the session**
Started by looking at your world differently; accept the risks and challenges and focus on developing the skills and resources to deal with them as they arise. On the floor: look at the ceiling—your world is different now.

Just one more challenge

We have become a cohesive group and we have shared a great deal of learning and fun. I think we should reward each other.

Shoulder massage

Fig. 9.11 Interactive workshop II

Short courses

The next two examples were short courses developed for presentation to general staff. As short courses, they were more formal, although discussion and group activities did occur. Each short course ran over two days and participants came from a wide range of employment settings.

Short course for women

Women in work: balancing the rightrope

Target group

Any woman who finds herself struggling to balance her personal roles and responsibilities with her work related requirements and expectations.

Course aims

Participants will have the opportunity to explore the way they currently function; to increase their awareness of their self-limiting behaviour; build confidence; learn practicel skills that can be applied in the work place and in personal situations; to empower them to be in better control of their lives.

Course objectives

Upon completion of this course participants should be able to:
- communicate assertively
- recognise your strengths and achievements
- express your needs and feelilngs positively
- recognise and reject unrealistic expectations
- plan strategies for manageable behaviour change
- harness the support of partners and colleagues.

Short course for managers

Making sense of staff education: the manager's guide

Target group

Managers without formal qualifications in education, who have a responsibility for staff development within their role and who need a practical approach to assist them to manage their responsibilities and get results.

Course aims

This course provides a practical explanation of the key components of staff education, from needs identification to the evaluation of results, with opportunities for individual application to the work situation.

Course objectives

Upon completion of this course participants should be able to:
- relate staff education to other staff management functions
- conduct a needs analysis
- identify and differentiate between categories of staff needs
- identify a range of possible strategies and resources
- develop a staff development plan
- design an evaluation tool to measure results.

Preparing for a presentation

Preparing for a presentation of any kind, speech, informal talk, or paper, requires careful consideration. This guide will assist you to plan any presentation. Note that the development of the introduction is presented at the end of the planning.

Preparing for a presentation
Organising your thoughts

- Brainstorm the main ideas: make a list of the points you want to cover.
- Develop the sub-points: what are the specific messages you wish to deliver?
- State the benefits: why people will want to hear what you have to say.
- Develop handouts: what information would you like people to take away with them and should this be in the form of a handout?
- Choose visual aids: what equipment or visual aids do you wish to use?
- Preview and review the three main points: Tell them what you are going to tell them — tell them — then tell them again.
- Develop the introduction.
- Develop the conclusion.

Feedback is the only true way to evaluate your performance. If you are really committed to improving your performance, you should invite participants to evalute your presentation. The following evaluation form will provide you with the information you need.

Presentation evaluation

Please make comments on the following aspects of my presentation. Please make constructive comments.

Voice and mannerisms ---

Organisation of material ---

Opening and closing --

The purpose: was it clear? ---

The use of visual aids --

Enthusiasm and conviction ---

What was the best part of the presentation? ------------------------------------

How could it be improved? ---

Resources

The following list of books and journals are identified as being particularly useful when working in staff development and education. Some of them have already been listed as references within chapters.

Books

Antonovsky A 1987 Unravelling the mystery of health: how people manage stress and stay healthy. Jossey-Bass, San Francisco

Davis M, Eshelman E R, McKay M 1988 The relaxation and stress reduction workbook. New Harbinger Publications, Oakland USA

Gardner H 1985 Frames of mind. Paladin, New York

Howard, R 1991 All about intelligence. New South Wales University Press, Sydney

Kroehnert G 1992 100 Training games. McGraw-Hill Book Company, Sydney

Malouf D 1990 How to create and deliver a dynamic presentation. Simon & Schuster, Australia

Navarra T, Lipkowitz, Navarra J G 1990 Therapeutic communication: a guide to effective interpersonal skills for health professionals. Slack, Thorofare, New Jersey

Stein-Parbury J 1993 Patient and person: developing interpersonal skills in nursing. Churchill Livingstone, Melbourne

Journals

The Australian Journal of Advanced Nursing. Australian Nursing Federation

Journal of Staff Development.

Contemporary Nurse: a Journal for the Australian Nursing Profession. Churchill Livingstone, Melbourne

Training and Development in Australia. Australian Institute of Training and Development

Collegian. Journal of Royal College of Nursing, Australia

Journal of Continuing Education in Nursing, USA

Music

The use of music to facilitate learning has been discussed in a number of places within this book. Examples of its use can also be seen within this chapter. The following list is given as a beginner's guide to the use of music.

Baroque music: background and relaxation music
Pachobel — The Canon; Vivaldi — Four Seasons; Bach — Brandenburg Concerto
Classical music: background and relaxation
Mozart — all compositions; Beethoven — Piano Concerto No.5; Symphony No. 9; Tchaikovsky — Sleeping Beauty; Brahms, Schuman, Rachmaninoff, Wagner — all compositions
Contemporary music: opening sessions; energisers
Zamfir — Music of the Pan Flute; Tina Turner — Simply the Best; Kenny G — Breathless
Relaxation music: meditation, learning facilitation
Tony O'Connor — all compositions

Index